The American Civil War Surgery Series

Edited by Ira M. Rutkow, M.D., Dr.P.H.

A MANUAL OF
MINOR SURGERY

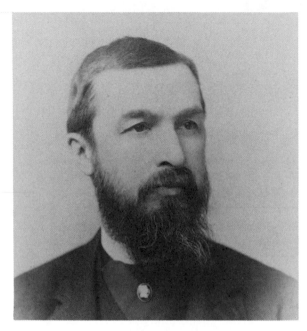

John Hooker Packard

1832–1907

National Library of Medicine

A MANUAL OF
MINOR SURGERY

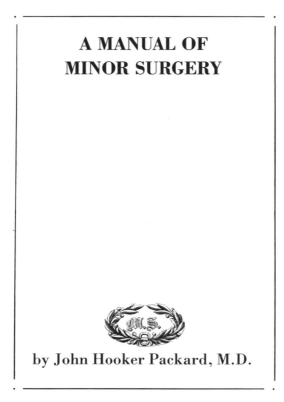

by John Hooker Packard, M.D.

Reprinted with a Biographical Introduction

by Ira M. Rutkow, M.D., Dr.P.H.

Norman Publishing

San Francisco

1990

Published by Norman Publishing
Division of Jeremy Norman & Co., Inc.
442 Post Street
San Francisco, California 94102-1579

Library of Congress Cataloging-in-Publication Data

Packard, John H. (John Hooker), 1832-1907.
A manual of minor surgery / by John Hooker Packard;
reprinted with a biographical introduction by Ira M. Rutkow.
p. cm. —(The American Civil War Surgery Series, No. 10)
Reprint. Originally published: Philadelphia: Lippincott, 1863.
ISBN 0-930405-08-0 (alk. paper)
1. Surgery, Minor—Handbooks, manuals, etc.
I. Rutkow, Ira M. II. Title. III. Series.
RD111.P25   1990   617'.024—dc19

The American Civil War Surgery Series, No. 10

This volume was reproduced from an original edition loaned
from the Francis A. Countway Library of Medicine, Boston.

This book is printed on acid-free paper, and its binding
materials have been chosen for strength and durability.

Manufactured in the United States of America.

John Hooker Packard

John Hooker Packard was born in Philadelphia on August 15, 1832, the son of Frederick A. Packard, a lawyer, and Elizabeth Dwight Hooker Packard. His ancestors were Puritans, and he was a direct descendant of the Reverend Thomas Hooker (1586–1647), one of the founders of Connecticut. Packard received most of his secondary education in the General Academic Department of the University of Pennsylvania during 1841–46. He received his undergraduate degree from that institution's department of arts in 1850 and an M.D. from its medical department in 1853.

In addition to his formal medical education, Packard had as a private preceptor the renowned anatomist Joseph Leidy (1823–91). Most of the skill in anatomical studies that Packard demonstrated throughout his life was the result of this early relationship with Leidy. From his youth, Packard had demonstrated considerable ability at drawing, and his patient histories and physical examinations were often filled with sketches. After graduating from medical school, Packard decided to study abroad and spent most of his time in Paris and London where he took courses in microscopy and regularly attended clinics at various hospitals.

In 1855 Packard returned to the United States, taking a position as resident physician at the Pennsylvania Hospital for eighteen months. While starting his own private practice, he held a clinical teaching position at the University of Pennsylvania, devoting himself particularly to anatomy, surgery, and obstetrics. He was said to have been quite popular as a teacher, but the only other academic position he ever held was a post as demonstrator of anatomy at the University of Pennsylvania in 1862–63.

Packard served in a number of capacities during the Civil War. He was initially appointed acting assistant surgeon in the United States Army, and was an attending surgeon to the Christian Street and Satterlee hospitals in Philadelphia. Packard was also consulting surgeon to the Haddington and Beverly army hospitals. During the Battle of Gettysburg, he received orders to report to the battlefield immediately. Although quite ill at the time from what later developed into typhoid fever, Packard worked in the field hospital for three days and nights until he was exhausted. He was then sent back to Philadelphia, but his military career was over.

In 1863 Packard was elected surgeon to the Episcopal Hospital in Philadelphia. He served in this capacity for twenty years, resigning when he was appointed surgeon at Pennsylvania Hospital in 1884. He held this position until retiring from active clinical practice in 1896. For a number of years he was also on the staff of St. Joseph's Hospital.

Packard was elected a fellow of the College of Physicians of Philadelphia in 1858 and served as its secretary from 1862 to 1877 and as vice-president from 1885 to 1888. He had the honor of delivering the first set of Mütter Lectures at that institution; these lectures were later published in book form as *Lectures on Inflammation* in 1865. Packard was also among the founders of the Philadelphia Academy of Surgery (1879), the Pathological Society of Philadelphia (of which he was president in 1867–68), and the Obstetrical Society of Philadelphia (of which he was president in 1877–78). In addition, Packard was one of the original founding members of the American Surgical Association (1880), serving as its elected treasurer from 1881 to 1884. He also found time to volunteer as an active member of the Pennsylvania Academy of the Fine Arts, and from 1884 until his death was on its Board of Directors.

Recognized for his expertise in the intricacies of medico-legal situations, Packard often served as a witness. He was a corresponding member of the New York Medico-Legal Society and in 1896 presented a paper before that group in which he suggested the use of a lethal gas chamber for the infliction of the death penalty. To cause asphyxiation, Packard proposed the extraction of oxygen from the atmosphere and the introduction of carbonic acid gas.

Packard was a prolific author. Among his books were *A Handbook of Operative Surgery* (1870) and *Sea-Air and Sea-Bathing* (1880). *The Manual of Minor Surgery* was published in one edition and served as a valuable adjunct to the other guides available to surgeons in the Union Army. Packard was also responsible for editing three editions of *The Philadelphia Medical Register and Directory* (1868, 1871, 1873). In 1859 he published a translation of *A Treatise on Fractures* by Joseph François Malgaigne (1806–65). From the second English edition of *A System of Surgery, Theoretical and Practical* by Timothy Holmes (1825–1907), Packard edited a three-volume American set, which was published in 1881–82. He also contributed to John Ashhurst's three-volume *International Encyclopedia of Surgery* (1881–86) by writing articles on poisoned wounds and injuries to bones—the latter a monograph of 260 pages. In addition, Packard wrote two chapters on colotomy and fractures and dislocations for John Marie Keating's (1852–1893) *Cyclopaedia of the Diseases of Children*.

In 1896 Packard infected himself during the course of a surgical operation, an accident that caused generalized sepsis. This so weakened him that he eventually was forced to give up all active medical work. Enforced idleness caused a depression that overshadowed the last ten years of his life. Packard succumbed to kidney failure brought on by cardiac insufficiency on May 21, 1907.

Packard was married to Elizabeth Wood on June 3, 1858. She was a niece of the renowned physician George Bacon Wood (1797–1879), who edited the monumental and authoritative *Dispensatory of the United States*. The Packards had six children, and two of his five sons became prominent physicians. Frederick A. Packard (1862–1902) was an internist and Francis R. Packard (1870–1950) was professor of diseases of the throat and nose at the University of Pennsylvania. Francis Packard was also a distinguished medical historian who wrote the comprehensive *History of Medicine in the United States* (1901), and edited the *Annals of Medical History* from its commencement in 1917 until its last volume in 1942.

A MANUAL

OF

MINOR SURGERY.

BY

JOHN H. PACKARD, M.D.,

DEMONSTRATOR OF ANATOMY IN THE UNIVERSITY OF PENNSYLVANIA, ONE OF THE
VISITING SURGEONS TO THE WEST PHILADELPHIA
MILITARY HOSPITAL, ETC. ETC.

WITH 145 ILLUSTRATIONS.

AUTHORIZED AND ADOPTED BY THE SURGEON-GENERAL OF THE
UNITED STATES ARMY FOR THE USE OF SURGEONS IN
THE FIELD AND GENERAL HOSPITALS.

PHILADELPHIA:

J. B. LIPPINCOTT & CO.

1863.

TO

GEORGE W. NORRIS, M.D.

IN HONOR OF HIS

DISTINGUISHED PROFESSIONAL STANDING,

AND

IN TOKEN OF GRATITUDE FOR

MANY KINDNESSES,

This little Volume is respectfully Inscribed

BY

THE AUTHOR.

PUBLISHERS' NOTICE.

THE Publishers of PACKARD'S MANUAL OF MINOR SURGERY are authorized to issue, for the information of the profession, the following Report of a Board, convened by order of the Surgeon-General, to examine the work with the view of its adoption for use in the Medical Department of the Army.

SURGEON-GENERAL'S OFFICE,
WASHINGTON CITY, D. C., MARCH 31st, 1863.

BRIG.-GEN. WM. A. HAMMOND,
SURGEON-GENERAL U. S. A.

General :—

The Board appointed to examine and report upon the merits of a work on *Minor Surgery*, submitted by Dr. John H. Packard, respectfully report that they have carefully examined this work, both in manuscript and in proof-sheets, and are satisfied that it is a better text-book upon the subject than any of the treatises with which the American market has hitherto been supplied.

J. H. BRINTON,
Surgeon U. S. Volunteers,
President of the Board.

J. J. WOODWARD,
Assistant-Surgeon, U. S. A.,
Recorder.

PREFACE.

THE aim kept in view in the preparation of the following pages has been to produce a practical manual; to put the reader in possession of clear directions for the ordinary duties (minor but not unimportant) of the practice of surgery. Some points belonging to the principles of the science have been necessarily touched upon; and a rigid critic might perhaps take exception to some of the matters introduced, as belonging to general and not to minor surgery. But here, as elsewhere in dealing with medical subjects, it is hard to draw a precise boundary-line, and better to overstep it than to fall short of it.

The author has endeavored in every case to present the best method of attaining the object sought, with such others as may afford desirable substitutes for it. Objectionable plans, or such as have deservedly fallen into disuse, have been either passed over in silence, or mentioned in the way of condemnation. Especial reference has always been had to such emergencies as constantly arise in civil as well as military practice.

Most of the cuts of instruments have been furnished by Mr. Kolbè, well known in this city as an able and ingenious manufacturer of surgical apparatus.   Many of the other illustrations are original.

In the earnest hope that it may be found useful, this little work is placed before the profession.

PHILADELPHIA, 1863,

TABLE OF CONTENTS.

A MANUAL

OF

MINOR SURGERY.

CHAPTER I.

THE POCKET-CASE, MATERIALS USED IN DRESSINGS, ETC.

BEFORE proceeding to the performance of even the slightest operation in surgery, everything that can possibly be required should be placed in readiness. Whether a wound is to be dressed, or a limb amputated, the surgeon should run over in his mind all the appliances he will need, all the exigencies that may arise; sponges, towels, dressings, ligatures, needles, instruments, all should be so arranged as to be at hand when called for. This is absolutely essential to the proper performance of every capital operation, and adds greatly to the comfort of all parties concerned in lesser surgical procedures.

¿ 1.—THE POCKET-CASE.

Some articles the surgeon should always carry with him, ready for use. They are put up in what is called the *pocket-case;* and are generally as follows: Scissors, a scalpel, bistouries, forceps, tenaculum, lancet, gum-lancet, needles, ligatures, porte-caustic, director, probes, and male and female catheter. Other instruments may be added, to any extent that the surgeon's fancy, or the peculiar demands of his practice, may dictate; but these are the commonly recognised essentials.*

A good pair of scissors is indispensable; some surgeons carry several, of different shapes, straight, curved on the flat, or bent at an angle at the joint. The best form is that last named, since it is never inconvenient, and sometimes answers when a plain straight pair would not. But they must be in good order; nothing looks so awkward as for the surgeon to have to *chew* a ligature or a suture-thread in two with dull scissors.

The scalpel is merely a knife with a convex cutting edge, that of a bistoury being always either straight or concave. A probe-pointed scalpel is of use in some operations. The bistouries are usually four in number, two curved and two straight; one of each pair being sharp-pointed, and the other ending in a probe or but-

---

* The instruments contained, according to the Army Regulations, (supply table last issued,) in the pocket-cases furnished to army medical officers, are as follows:—

One scalpel.	One tenaculum.
Three bistouries.	One scissors.
One tenotome.	One director.
One gum-lancet.	Three probes.
Two thumb-lancets.	One caustic-holder.
One razor, small.	One silver catheter, compound.
One artery-forceps.	
One dressing-forceps.	Six yards suture-wire, iron.
One artery-needle.	$\frac{1}{4}$ ounce ligature-silk.
Six surgeon's needles.	$\frac{1}{8}$ ounce wax.

ton-point. The handles of these knives are usually
made of plain tortoise-shell or buffalo-horn; and a
small slide, to keep the blades firm when shut or open,
is provided. Space is sometimes economized by combining two blades in one handle; but this plan is a bad
one, unless very great care is taken to clean both blades
whenever either one is used.

Fig. 1.   Fig. 2.   Fig. 3.

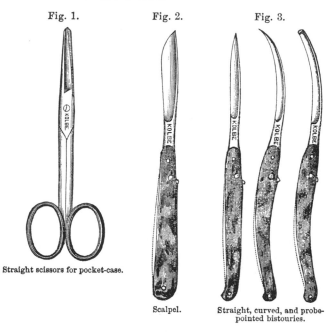

Straight scissors for pocket-case.

Scalpel.   Straight, curved, and probe-
pointed bistouries.

The forceps supplied are usually of two kinds; the
polypus or dressing-forceps, and the artery-forceps.
The former are shaped much like scissors, with ring-
handles, and blades filed with transverse ridges, so as
to afford a good hold of any object grasped between
them. The latter are like the ordinary dissecting

forceps, except that they have a slide, to keep them
shut when necessary, and each branch has a longitudinal groove at the inner side of its extremity, shaped

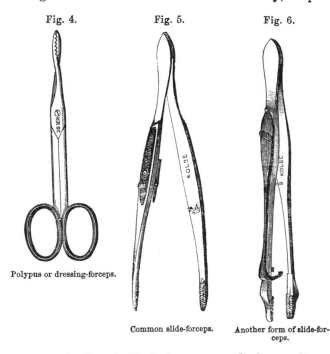

Fig. 4.   Fig. 5.   Fig. 6.

Polypus or dressing-forceps.

Common slide-forceps.   Another form of slide-forceps.

so as to take firm hold of the upper end of a needle or
hare-lip pin.

About the tenaculum, the only peculiarity is that it
is placed in a handle, like one of the knives, and has a
slide to keep it immovable when shut up or open.   The
same may be said of the gum-lancet.

The lancet is simply a common thumb-lancet.   If
the surgeon has himself to do any bleeding that may be
required in his practice, he should keep one lancet for

this purpose, and another for vaccination. The needles, director, and probes vary with the ideas of the surgeon. It is better that the director and probes should be of pure silver, so that no degree of bending will injure them. Among the probes may be placed the *porte-mêche*, for substituting the finger in carrying a ligature or small tampon into any place too deep and narrow to allow convenient entrance to the finger. It is merely a piece of wire about the size of a probe, having at one end a sort of minute fork. (See *Fig.* 10.) It is often

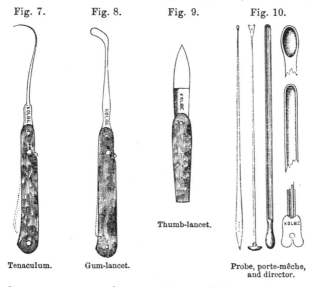

Fig. 7.   Fig. 8.   Fig. 9.   Fig. 10.

Thumb-lancet.

Tenaculum.   Gum-lancet.   Probe, porte-mêche, and director.

of very great use in operations. Various shapes and sizes of needles should be kept to suit different cases; and a supply of silk thread, silver, iron, and lead-wire for sutures should be kept. Ligatures are made of silk thread.

The shaft of the catheter is provided with a screw-thread towards its lower end, fitting either of two tips,

Fig. 11.

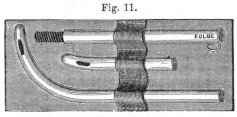

Catheter for pocket-case.   Showing the shaft with two tips; one for
use in the male and the other in the female subject.

one long, and curved so as to suit the male urethra, the
other short and bent slightly, for the female.

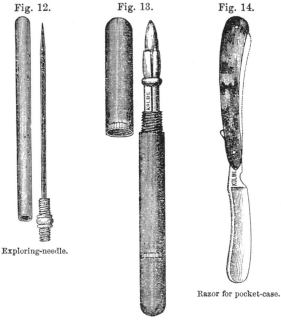

Fig. 12.   Fig. 13.   Fig. 14.

Exploring-needle.

Porte-caustic.

Razor for pocket-case.

Another instrument often supplied in the pocket-case

is the grooved exploring-needle, with a handle made to serve as a sheath when the needle is not in use. Cases rarely occur, however, in which the employment of this instrument is necessary or even proper; and much harm may be done with it.

The porte-caustic is made of silver, ebony, or hard-rubber. Its tip, which grasps the caustic, should be composed of platinum, so as to undergo no chemical change; and the instrument is generally arranged so that by screwing one of its parts upon another it may be very much lengthened, for the purpose of touching the os uteri, pharynx, etc. A razor kept in the pocket-case will sometimes be found of use, in shaving a part to be operated on or dressed.

§ 2.—THE DRESSING-BOX

Is essential to order and comfort in hospital surgery. It is simply a wooden box with a handle, like a large knife-tray, in which is kept a supply of bandages, lint, charpie, ligatures, sponges, strips of adhesive plaster of various widths, towels, a pair of large scissors, a well-furnished pin-cushion, and whatever else the surgeon is likely to need as he makes his rounds. It ought to be divided into compartments, and kept always in order and well replenished. Besides the articles already mentioned, it should contain a few gum-catheters and bougies, with some oil or lard for anointing them; some cerate and a spatula; a bottle or cup of common whiskey for washing, and another of spirit of turpentine. Another instrument which will sometimes be of use is a large double probe, commonly called a gunshot-probe.

The nurse or some other attendant carries the dressing-box round after the surgeon as he makes his visit.

§ 3.—THE MATERIALS, ETC. EMPLOYED IN DRESSINGS.

Although in an emergency we may make use of almost any material for surgical dressings, yet there are certain articles especially adapted for the purpose, which call for a brief enumeration. Properly speaking, this list should include splints, styptics, etc.; but these may be more conveniently described elsewhere.

LINT is more useful than anything else would be, for certain purposes. It may be readily made by drawing out all the cross threads from a piece of old linen, leaving only enough to hold the other threads together; its fineness will be in proportion to that of the stuff. A very fine form of it, suitable for small wounds, is made by scraping one side of an old piece of linen with a blunt table-knife. "Patent lint," made by a machine, is sold in the shops; it comes in various grades of fineness, either in long pieces or in pound bundles. One of its surfaces is smooth, the other is covered with a cotton-like down. Its expensiveness is the only objection to it.

Lint may be employed either in making compresses, as a means of applying ointments or lotions to a part, or as a dry dressing. Generally speaking, its smooth side should be next the affected surface. Nothing can be simpler than the making of a compress, the only points to be regarded being its adaptation to the shape of the part, and the regulation of its thickness. By suitable folding, a piece of lint or old linen may be fitted or *graduated* so as to press evenly upon a quite irregular surface. The *perforated* compress is made by folding the stuff so that it acquires a considerable thickness, and then cutting out a portion so as to fit any part which needs protection from pressure; it is in this way that the India-rubber air-pads sold in the shops are useful in preventing bed-sores, since when inflated they form a circular compress upon which the body rests, while the sacrum is raised and free in the open space at the centre. The *cribriform* compress is provided with apertures in greater or less number, through which discharges may escape to be absorbed by charpie or some other material, arranged upon its outer surface. The Maltese cross is made by folding a square piece of stuff into a triangle, folding this again in the same manner, and then cutting away the two *folded* edges to near their point of junction; on opening out the piece, it will be found to have assumed the well-known form indicated by the above name. A little practice will enable one to judge quite accurately how large the square should be, and how much should be cut away at the angles. This form of compress is much used for stumps, as well as in affections of the female breast.

CHARPIE is composed of the separated threads of linen fabrics; its coarseness or fineness will obviously depend on that of the original stuff. The threads are generally tangled up, so as to form a porous mass. Cotton threads are sometimes used, but are more heating to the part than those of flax.

Charpie is mainly used as a means of absorbing discharges; with this view it may be very advantageously employed in the dressing of stumps, abscesses, or sup-

purating wounds. It should never be placed in immediate contact with the affected surface, unless previously
soaked or anointed. Authors describe various forms in
which charpie may be employed,—the plumasseau or
pledget, the roll, the tent, the mesh, the pellet, the tampon, etc. But these differ only in their shape, not in
the object of their employment, and may be easily devised to suit the occasion; it is therefore unnecessary
to enter into detail here with respect to them.

RAW COTTON, as sold in rolls in the shops, is often
used for the padding of splints, or to protect parts especially exposed to pressure. It is also extensively used
as an application to burns, when the cuticle is not removed; and in such cases acts admirably. It is employed as a very gentle irritant to the skin, in cases of
rheumatism, and to envelop a part of which the temperature is lowered, as by the tying of a large artery;
being retained in place by means of a loosely-applied
roller.

BRAN, although its use has been hitherto mainly confined to the treatment of compound fractures, may be
very suitably employed in many cases of injury of the
soft tissues. It is simply heaped over the affected part,
and acts by excluding the air, absorbing discharges,
and preventing flies from depositing their eggs in the
wound, so as to breed maggots. Nothing can serve the
purpose better, in the heat of summer, than this light,
cool, and cleanly dressing; while the soiled portions can
be removed with the greatest ease, without the slightest
disturbance of the limb.

Tow sometimes answers very well to protect the patient's bed, by absorbing discharges; but it is too coarse and irritating to be applied directly to the surface of the body.

Sponge-tent, an article at present almost out of date, is made by soaking pieces of sponge in melted beeswax; it is cut and moulded to the required size and shape, and then introduced wherever the union of opposed surfaces is undesirable, or where distension of a passage is to be effected or kept up. It is very irritating, and not very cleanly.

Adhesive Plaster, the *Emplastrum Resinæ* of the U. S. Pharmacopœia, is an article familiar to every one. It is merely lead plaster, with the addition of some resin, one part to six, spread upon one surface of thin muslin. It may be used for keeping the lips of a wound in contact; for making compression, as in inflammation of the testicle or in ulceration of the leg, according to rules elsewhere given; for making extension and counter-extension in certain fractures, as will be mentioned when we come to speak of that class of injuries; and in a great many other cases.

Adhesive plaster is very irritating, and should never be applied as a mere covering to wounds or sores; its traction should be exerted only upon the sound skin. Hence it is always cut into strips for use; and the width of the piece as sold is such that the strips may for almost every purpose be cut crosswise. The end of the piece should be towards the surgeon's left, and the edge opposite him held by an assistant; then he makes the other edge tense, by taking hold of its extremity with

the finger and thumb of his left hand, the thumb uppermost, and stretching it by means of the middle and ring
fingers of the same hand; now passing one blade of a
pair of scissors underneath the edge, he carries them
straight across by a quick pushing motion.　Each successive strip is cut from the extremity of the piece in
the same way; but when the length required is such
that this would involve much waste in the subsequent
application, the strips may be cut along the piece instead of across it.

Fig. 15.

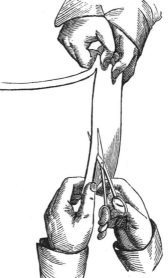

The strips thus cut must be warmed for use, unless
the temperature of the air is so high as to render them
sufficiently adhesive.　A very good plan is to have a
can of hot water, to the outside of which the back of

each strip is applied before it is put on; some surgeons prefer the flame of a spirit-lamp. Friction of the strip by drawing it several times between the thumb and finger, in the absence of other sources of heat, may answer the same purpose, and is more convenient when but a few strips are to be employed.

In order to remove adhesive plaster, all that is necessary is to sponge it either with hot water, which softens the adhesive material, or with oil of turpentine, which dissolves it. Perhaps I need hardly remark that hairy parts should be shaved before the plaster is applied, not only because it will hold better, but because its subsequent removal is much easier if this is done. Some other points will be alluded to in connection with the dressing of wounds.

In order to prevent the adhesive strips from stretching after they are applied, they are either stretched as much as possible by the surgeon before they are put on, or, which is better, they are cut in the direction of the length instead of the breadth of the piece.

ISINGLASS PLASTER is sold at present at all the apothecary shops, and has a very extensive popularity. It is made by washing over one side of a piece of thin silk with a spirituous solution of isinglass; and is generally used just as adhesive plaster is, except that it is moistened with a wet sponge instead of being heated, in order to its application. Being quite mild and unirritating, it may be employed as an artificial scab for small ulcers.

For use on the field, in military surgery, isinglass plaster has some very great advantages over the ordinary resin plaster. Its bulk is less, and in warm climates and seasons it may be carried without undergoing any change. The water required to prepare it for instant application can always be had, and dressings may be performed very rapidly with it. Hence it has obtained great favor with our army surgeons during the present war.

When neither of these forms of adhesive plaster can be obtained, a good substitute may be made by mixing flour with white of eggs, so as to form a paste. Strips of thin linen or muslin imbued with this and laid on the skin, will in drying take a very firm hold. Wetting with warm water will loosen them again.

COLLODION, made by dissolving gun-cotton in sulphuric ether, is much used as an adhesive material. After operations on the eye, it is employed to keep the lids closed. For this purpose, or for keeping the lips of a wound in apposition, a piece of fine soft rag is laid with its centre directly over the affected part, and then the collodion is painted on with a camel's-hair pencil, so as to attach each end of the rag to the sound skin beneath it. Thus the wound or the eye is left free from irritation, or may have any other suitable dressing confined upon it. Small wounds may be simply painted over with the collodion, which is also applied in some cases for the sake of the contraction undergone by it in drying; small nævi may sometimes be entirely discussed in this way, and occasionally even vascular engorgements of the testicle, breast and other organs.

Mr. Hubbell, the well-known druggist of this city, prepares a non-contractile form of collodion, by adding to every ʒj ʒss of liquid Venice turpentine or of castor oil. The former makes a better preparation, unless it is specially desirable to avoid irritating the parts. Either will be found to possess advantages over collodion as commonly prepared.

An excellent substitute for blisters of the ordinary form is obtained by dissolving an ethereal extract of cantharides in collodion. It is called *blistering* or *cantharidal collodion;* the mode of employing it being simply to paint it over the desired extent of surface by means of a camel's-hair pencil. Its action is hastened by laying over it a piece of oiled silk, so as to prevent the evaporation of the ether. Some surgeons also use collodion as a vehicle for the application of creosote, in cases of erysipelas or erythema of the traumatic variety.

Whenever it is desirable to remove collodion, either simple or medicated, this may readily be done by dissolving it away with ether.

WATER-GLASS is the name given to an article lately proposed by Küchenmeister as a partial substitute for collodion. It is made by melting together 10 parts of potassa, 15 of powdered quartz, and 1 of charcoal, forming a blackish-gray mass; this is dissolved in 5 parts of water, and the solution evaporated to a semi-fluid consistence. The substance thus formed has an alkaline reaction, and dries slowly, forming an impermeable coating to wounds, swellings, and skin diseases; on account of its alkaline reaction, it is particularly recommended for the stings of insects, snake-bites, etc. As yet, however, it has been tried only to a very limited extent.

POULTICES or CATAPLASMS, if well made, are extremely useful; they are intended to act mainly by their heat and moisture, except in some cases, when they are applied cold, and renewed as fast as they acquire heat from the part. These *refrigerant* poultices are not, however, in very common use, the cold water-dressing answering much the same purpose.

Very various materials are employed in the making of dressings of this kind. Flaxseed meal is perhaps the best, but rye meal, Indian meal, and bread, are also suitable. Slippery-elm bark contains a great deal of mucilage, and hence forms a good emollient. Any of these substances may be worked into a semi-solid mass with water.

Sometimes it is desirable to medicate poultices, with a view to relieve some special condition of the affected part. This may be done by modifying either their solid or their liquid ingredients. If an anodyne effect is to be sought, we may either incorporate a little watery extract of opium with the mass of a flaxseed poultice, or add some laudanum to the water used in mixing it. Or hops may be substituted for the flaxseed; bruised poppy-heads are sometimes used in the same way.

Fermenting poultices are much used in cases of gangrene, unhealthy ulcers, etc. They are made by mixing up Indian meal with yeast or porter. When the odor of a diseased part is offensive, it may be corrected by adding very finely pulverized charcoal or burnt coffee to the other ingredients of a poultice, or by putting a little solution of chlorinated soda, or some other disinfecting fluid, into the water used for mixing up the mass. (See *Disinfectants.*)

Astringent and stimulating poultices are sometimes employed to excite action in an indolent ulcer, cavity, or sinus; they may be made by simply adding to the

ordinary poultice some article having the desired property. Sometimes, however, the basis of the mass is
changed; thus white-oak bark, macerated in water,
makes a very good astringent poultice for indolent
ulcers on the leg, while for some affections of the eye
an analogous preparation is found in the curd formed
by the action of alum upon the white of eggs, or upon
milk.

In order that a poultice may be efficient or even
endurable, certain rules must be observed in the making
and application of it. The mass being duly mixed, free
from lumps, neither too stiff nor too thin, should be
evenly spread upon a piece of soft linen or muslin, in a
layer of suitable extent and thickness. All round the
edges of the piece a margin of about an inch should be
left uncovered, to be folded over so as to prevent the
escape of portions of the mass. Some writers advise
that the poultice should be placed between two layers of
thin muslin, others that its surface should be covered
with a piece of thin gauze, and others again that a few
drops of sweet oil or a little lard should be smeared
over it; the object being to provide against the adhesion of the poultice, or of portions of it, to the skin.
The latter of these plans is very simple and convenient,
in ordinary cases; but some poultices, such as those
made of hops or of Indian meal, have so little cohesion
that it is better to cover them over. Outside of the
stuff upon which the poultice is spread, a piece of oiled
silk should be laid, an inch larger every way; this
serves to confine the moisture and warmth, and to
prevent discomfort from the soaking outward of the
liquid portion of the mass. Any convenient means may

3*

be employed for keeping the dressing so arranged in position.

Once in twenty-four hours, or oftener if it seems necessary, the poultice may be renewed; a fresh one being prepared before the one last put on is disturbed.

WATER-DRESSINGS may be either cold or warm, simple or medicated. Many surgeons make use of them almost exclusively, on account of their simplicity and cleanliness; while their ready accessibility often gives them great value as temporary expedients, even where other means are to be permanently employed. The effect of water externally applied is not necessarily confined to the surface, since it is a physiological fact that the skin takes it up by absorption. Hence, in inflammation, the blood contained in the vessels of the part will be diluted, and perhaps in this way the chemical processes involved may be rendered less active. Moreover, any medicinal substance dissolved in the water will be carried in also; such as are merely mixed or suspended in it will of course act upon the surface alone. It may be well also to observe here, that when the article in solution is in any degree astringent or stimulating, its action upon the deeper seated tissues will be more apt to be efficient if the proportion of it is small than if it is large; since in the latter case its agency upon the superficial vessels may be so powerful as to prevent its passing through them. Lint, or any soft absorbent fabric may be used for the purpose of maintaining the liquid in contact with the part; irrigation may in some cases be substituted for this method, but is much more troublesome and difficult of arrangement, so that its application is less general.

Cold water acts by depressing the vital force of the part, and perhaps also by inducing contraction of the non-striated muscular fibres which enter into the structure of the skin. It should be as cold as the patient can bear with comfort, and needs renewal as often as its temperature rises by the abstraction of heat from the part. Hence it should not only be allowed to evaporate freely, but should be applied by means of a thin layer of whatever fabric is used, so that the portion next the skin may not accumulate warmth. Ice-water is a most excellent application in many cases, especially to compound fractures, gunshot wounds, wounds of joints, and wounds of the head. My own plan is to place old linen rags, soaked in ice-water, upon the part, and then to lay one or more small lumps of ice, folded up in another wet rag, upon the top; in this way the temperature is kept down. Prof. Esmarch, of Kiel, has been the most prominent advocate of cold dressings in surgery.

Astringents, anodynes, and refrigerants, — such as tannin, acetate of lead, watery extract of opium, etc., —may be combined with cold water. Sometimes demulcents, such as slippery-elm bark, sassafras pith, or bran, may be added with advantage.

When irrigation is thought desirable, it may be employed by means of a tube arranged to act as a syphon, a bucket or other vessel containing the cold water being placed at a convenient height, and a piece of lint or of any other suitable fabric being placed upon the part so as to spread the liquid over it. A piece of India-rubber cloth or oiled silk should be laid so as to conduct the waste water off without any risk of the bed or bedclothes becoming wet. If the affected part is of any extent, a tube of suitable length, perforated with holes, may be suspended over it, and the water turned on by means of a stop-cock. Or if the part be small, an article like the *rose* of a watering-pot may be substituted for the tube.

Warm water has of itself a soothing and relaxing influence upon any part to which it is applied. Lint or any other soft fabric may be used as a vehicle for it; and as any evaporation would lower its temperature, a piece of oiled silk or of thin India-rubber cloth must always be placed over it, just as in the case of the poultice. An article called *spongio-piline* was brought forward in London some years ago, intended to supply the place of both lint and oiled silk in the application of the warm water-dressing. One of its surfaces, soft and absorbent, receives the water and is placed next the skin; the other, smooth and water-proof, serves to prevent evaporation. Although a very neat and elegant contrivance, this material cannot, for obvious reasons, be used to any great extent; the cost of it alone would be an item of some moment, since the same piece could very seldom be used more than once. Many surgeons discard the poultice entirely, preferring to use warm water; but in fact there is often a good deal of room for choice between the two.

Warm water is much more frequently medicated than cold, principally because it requires less constant renewal. Astringents, such as sulphate of zinc or copper, chloride of zinc, tannic acid, etc. etc., may be dissolved in it. Deodorants—creosote, chloride of soda, permanganate of potash, etc.—may be added to it in greater or less proportion for the dressing of offensive sores. Demulcents are often combined with it, and increase its soothing and relaxing effect.

The substance known as *oakum*, which is simply a mass of the separated shreds of old tarred rope, when well soaked in hot water, constitutes a very cheap form of wet dressing. It is slightly astringent, and the quantity of tar contained in it, although small, is sufficient to give it an antiseptic property. When applied to an ulcer or granulating sore, it should be covered with oiled silk just as wet lint is, and changed as often as circumstances may seem to require. Oakum has lately been introduced extensively in the United States army, and has long been popular with some of our naval surgeons.

Ointments and *cerates* are less used of late years than they formerly were, wet dressings having taken their place in a very great degree. They are of different kinds according to the end desired in their application.

Lard with all the salt washed out of it is a very mild and unirritating ointment for burns and ulcers. Castor oil, and the fine sweet oil sold for table use may also be employed. Some surgeons consider a combination of castor oil with glycerin as an excellent dressing. The simple cerate of the U. S. Pharmacopœia is also very bland.

Of irritating and stimulant ointments we have a very large variety. Blistering cerate (ceratum cantharidis), tartar emetic ointment, resin ointment (which by the addition of oil of turpentine constitutes Kentish's ointment), savin cerate, and many others, are well known.

Astringent ointments and cerates are made by adding the watery extract of galls, the oxide of zinc, and other astringent articles, to lard or simple cerate.

Anodyne ointments are composed of one or more narcotic extracts incorporated in the same way.

Tin-foil and *sheet-lead* may be used as a dressing to ulcers in very many cases. They act simply by protecting the surface. Not being, like cerates, capable of becoming rancid, these articles possess great value. My own experience with them has been highly favorable to their use.

Tin-foil is not composed of the pure metal, some zinc and antimony being added to prevent brittleness; it therefore suits those cases best which call for a stimulating treatment. After it has been applied to an ulcer for a few days, it causes pain, and the granulations become exuberant. Sheet-lead contains no admixture, and is less irritating.

On the score of economy, these articles claim attention, and are strongly recommended to the notice of practitioners. A piece of either substance is cut out as nearly as may be in the shape of the sore to be covered, and being laid in place, is confined by means of adhesive strips. Some absorbent material should be added outside of the metal, to take up the discharges as they escape. This plan, I repeat, has afforded me the best results.

CHAPTER II.

OF THE APPLICATION OF DRESSINGS.

The labor of the surgeon, especially in a large hospital, will be much lessened by the observance of method in all his dressings; while the sufferings of his patients will be in an inverse ratio to his system, dexterity, and care.

Before exposing the injured or diseased part, the surgeon should place his patient in such a position that he and his assistants can do what is necessary without hindrance.

All the dressings to be applied should be made ready, or at least the materials for them; sponges, basins of warm water, Castile soap, and towels are wanted in almost every case, and should be placed at hand. The part must be steadily supported, by one or more assistants if necessary, while the surgeon proceeds to remove the old dressings, to cleanse the surface, and to dress it afresh.

During the dressing, the bed, clothes, etc. should be protected by water-proof cloths, or by holding the part so that all discharges, and the water used in washing, may flow either into the receptacle for the soiled dressings or into the basin; the latter plan is better.

When, as in some amputations, the removal of all the adhesive strips would endanger the falling apart of the lips of the wound, they should be replaced by new ones as they are successively taken off. It is always proper, in order to obviate the risk of drawing the wound open, to lift the strip from each end towards the middle. (See Fig. 16.)

In all cases, the first aim of the surgeon should be to promote the welfare of his patient; and this sometimes requires some sacrifice of appearances. It is never to be forgotten in putting on a dressing, that it must at some time be taken off; for instance, it is bad surgery

Fig. 16.

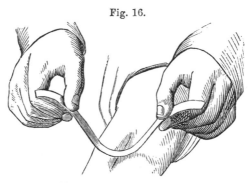

Mode of removal of adhesive strips.

to wind a strip of adhesive plaster round and round a part, so that its end cannot be readily found for removal.

SPECIAL DRESSINGS.—There are some dressings for special purposes, which can be best described here.

(1) *Of the Dressing of Stumps.*—After the removal of a limb, hæmorrhage having completely ceased, the wound is closed by bringing the opposite edges of the skin together. The ends of the ligatures are brought outside, sometimes all at one end, sometimes in two bundles, one at each end, of the wound; and a sufficient

number of points of the interrupted suture, either silken or metallic, are applied to keep the edges in close apposition. Some surgeons, among whom is Mr. Teale, of London, whose method of amputation by rectangular flaps is so well known, are in favor of leaving the stump without any further dressing, merely supporting the bedclothes over it. Generally, however, the sutures are reinforced by a sufficient number of adhesive strips, placed at suitable intervals, and long enough to take a firm hold. Over this a piece of lint or soft rag, anointed with cerate of some unirritating kind, (fresh lard is as good as anything,) is laid; it should be shaped so as to lie smoothly and without folds, which may be done by cutting it out square, applying it over the face of

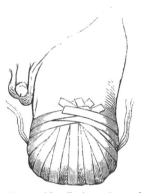

Fig. 17.

Stump with adhesive strips applied. The ligatures are seen in a bundle at either side.

the stump, and then pinching up folds and snipping them away until the surface is fitted. A thin layer of charpie being placed over this, a roller may now be applied, beginning well up on the limb, and surrounding it firmly until near enough to the wound, when recurrent turns are made over the face of the stump, as directed in the chapter on Bandages. This plan of dressing is particularly useful when patients have to be removed soon after the operation, as sometimes happens in military practice.

Some surgeons simply place a cold water-dressing on

the stump, over the adhesive strips. Some prefer warm water. Others again use astringent solutions.

Should no bleeding occur, and the stump remain comfortable, there is no need for removing the dressings for several days, unless they become disordered, when they must be reapplied.

In taking them off, the turns of the bandage should be cut along the upper surface of the stump, with a pair of blunt-pointed *bandage-scissors.* (See Chap. VI.) The cerate, etc. and the divided portions of bandage may then be turned down, softening them if need be with some warm water, without any derangement of the stump. A careful assistant, standing or sitting on the edge of the bed, with his back towards the patient, now lifts up and supports the stump in both hands, while the surgeon takes off each strip successively and replaces it with a new one; the portion of the strip crossing the wound being invariably the last removed, as before mentioned. (See *Fig.* 16.)

Suppuration having been established, the dressings must be renewed daily. After about a week, the sutures may be cut and withdrawn. Very gentle traction may be made on the smaller ligatures, at about the tenth day, should they not come away earlier of themselves. The adhesive strips should be employed until the wound has quite firmly healed, and after that a recurrent bandage or a cap fitted to the stump is useful as a protection. Several months should be allowed to elapse before an artificial limb is thought of.

(2) *Of the dressing of accidental wounds.* Certain general principles obtain in regard to all wounds, of whatever character and in whatever part of the body. These are :

1. To arrest hæmorrhage.

2. To cleanse the wound and remove foreign bodies.

3. To promote healing, with as little deformity as possible.

4. To keep down inflammation.

We have now to consider the application of these principles to the dressing of *incised, contused, lacerated,* and *gunshot* wounds of the various regions; the other varieties, *punctured, penetrating* and *poisoned* wounds, deriving their interest and importance, as well as the rules for their treatment, from circumstances beyond the scope of the present work.

Incised wounds, or clean cuts, are apt to be attended with hæmorrhage, the methods of checking which are elsewhere detailed. (See Chapter III.) As a temporary resource, the artery supplying the part may be pressed upon, by means of a tourniquet, a Spanish windlass,* or a bandage and compress. The latter means will

Fig. 18.

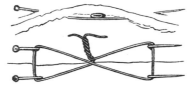

Modification of the twisted suture, employed by the author!

often be amply sufficient for the permanent arrest of bleeding from scalp-wounds. If a small or medium-

---

* Pressure by these means would at first *increase* the flow of blood, by impeding the venous current.

sized vessel is divided in the skin, one of the sutures may be made to transfix both its cardiac and distal end; or Prof. Simpson's plan of acupressure may be resorted to, a ligature being then twisted round the ends of the needles. (See *Fig*. 18.) Larger vessels may be safely dealt with in this latter method, especially if there is any difficulty about isolating them for the purpose of applying a ligature.

Let it be borne in mind that the more complete the arrest of the bleeding, the better the chance of speedy adhesion between the divided surfaces.

Healing is promoted by accurate adaptation of the edges of the wound, and by placing the part at perfect rest, on a splint if necessary, in such a position as to relax the muscles. This end is also answered by preventing or allaying inflammation, by means of cold or ice-water.

It should not be forgotten that separated parts, such as the ear, nose, or tip of the finger, may be made to unite if accurately replaced before they are actually dead; and therefore that attempts should be made at such reposition if the smallest chance of success is present.

Contusions are almost invariably attended with ecchymosis, swelling and pain; they sometimes terminate in abscess.

Much relief is afforded by the early application of leeches, followed by that of cold or ice-water, to which may be added lead-water and laudanum if the pain is severe,—say f℥j of each to f℥vj of water. At a later stage, gentle frictions with whiskey, with laudanum or chloroform and sweet oil, (one part to two,) or with the hand alone, will be found of advantage.

Lacerated wounds, even when severe and extensive,

are less apt than incised to be followed by serious hæmorrhage. But they are generally more difficult of coaptation, and there is often a tendency to sloughing of their edges which gives trouble. Suppuration almost necessarily occurs in them.

Sutures are usually inadmissible here. Adhesive strips, of resin or isinglass-plaster, not very tensely applied, may prevent somewhat the gaping of the wound, which should be very thoroughly cleansed. Cold or ice-water is generally the best dressing, but warm water should be substituted if it gives the patient greater ease.

Gunshot wounds are of especial importance and interest to the army surgeon. They have, as remarked by John Bell, "a peculiarity, but no mystery;" no other agency having so great force in so small a compass.

The hæmorrhage from recent gunshot wounds is seldom dangerous, unless a large artery is partially cut across, so that it cannot retract, or unless the ball is moving so rapidly that its effects on the tissues are like those of a knife. Life would be destroyed by complete division in this way of the carotid or femoral, or even of smaller vessels, unless the flow of blood be at once arrested. When profuse bleeding does occur upon the receipt of the wound, and especially if the patient has to undergo transportation, the rule given by Prof. Longmore* is imperative; the artery must be found and tied. Should the seat of the injury be such as to render this procedure difficult or dangerous, ligation of the trunk higher up, in the usual way, would be called for. The tourniquet cannot safely be trusted to. In military practice, attendants on the wounded in the field or hos-

---

* On Gunshot Wounds, p. 52.

4*

Fig. 19.

pital should always be instructed, in cases of hæmorrhage, to apply a finger over the spot whence the blood is seen to issue, until further measures can be adopted by the medical officer.

Secondary hæmorrhage, an artery giving way by ulceration or sloughing, is much more common. It is most apt to occur between the fifth and twelfth days; but I have reported a case* in which it came on fifty-six days after a gunshot wound of the thigh, the ball having lodged in the limb. Temporarily, the tourniquet may be employed, but ligation of the vessel of supply, or amputation, will usually be rendered necessary in these cases.

The cleansing of the wound and removal of foreign bodies, in this class of injuries, can hardly be too carefully attended to. Whenever possible, the finger should be used instead of a probe for the detection of matters which have lodged, the wound being somewhat enlarged if necessary. A very large gunshot or ball-probe may be used when the presence of a ball is suspected, or to determine whether or not a bone has been shattered; but the finger has the great advantage of being able to detect bits of clothing, etc., which would give no special sensation to the fingers through a probe.

Before making this examination, the part injured should be placed as nearly as possible in the exact position in which it was when struck. If a probe has to be employed, it should be

Gunshot or
ball-probe.

* Am. Journal of the Med. Sciences, July, 1857.

curved or bent as much as may by trial be found necessary to enable it to follow the track of the ball. The
utmost gentleness should be observed in all this explo-
ration; and care should be taken to support the part so
that the tissues may not yield before the probe or finger.

Should the ball, a piece of shell, or any foreign body,
be distinctly felt under the skin at a distance from its
point of entry, the proper plan is for the surgeon to
secure it in this position by suitable pressure on the
circumjacent skin, and then to cut down upon and remove it; the cut so made being called a *counter-
opening*.

When, however, the foreign body lies so near its
point of entry that it can be readily reached, some
form of bullet-extractor must be used. Much ingenuity
has been expended in the invention of instruments of
this kind; but after all, skill in the hand of the operator
is the essential point.

Often a simple scoop, such as is placed at the upper
extremity of the grooved director, may be made to engage the foreign body, so as to draw it out. A somewhat
more complicated instrument is made on the same principle as the *curette articulée* (for the urethra) of Leroy
d'Etiolles, which is like a straight director in shape, but
has a joint near one extremity so arranged as to be bent
to any desired angle up to 90° by the turning of a screw
at the other end. This, being introduced straight, is
passed alongside of the ball or other foreign body, and
then bent beyond it so as to engage it for removal.
The mechanism of this is the same as that of the double
forceps shown in *Fig.* 21. Another extractor, known
in this city as Levis's, but of doubtful parentage, consists of a tube with a recurved extremity, against which

a shaft, sliding in the tube and ending in a point, can be pushed down. The modus operandi of this instrument can be readily seen, but it is also evident that it is

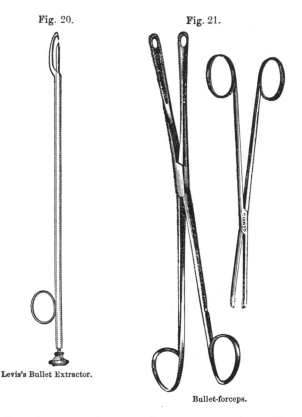

Fig. 20.   Fig. 21.

Levis's Bullet Extractor.

Bullet-forceps.

adapted to very few cases in actual practice. Forceps of various shapes will be found useful as extractors; the ordinary dressing or polypus-forceps are sometimes employed to advantage, as well as the slide-forceps of the pocket-case. Another form is shown in *Fig.* 21.

Everett's forceps are so made that one blade fits into
the other, so that both are introduced like the common
scoop, when by a rotation of the handles they are

Fig. 22.   Fig. 23.

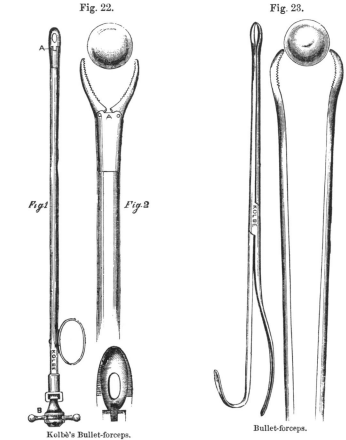

Fig 1   *Fig 2*

Kolbè's Bullet-forceps.   Bullet-forceps.

brought into opposition; they can then be separated
and the ball grasped. Still another form is so made as
to be passed in closed, like a probe, *Fig.* 22, 1, when the

turning of a screw at the other end separates the blades, which are short and strong, *Fig.* 22, 2; the ball or other foreign body being caught between these, they are made to grasp it by turning the screw the other way, and are then drawn out.* The extractors with a screw, intended to penetrate and thus take hold of the ball, are now generally abandoned. Should the bullet be lodged in a bone, the use of an elevator or lever may be called for to pry it out of its seat.

The wound being thus, if possible, cleared of foreign bodies, is now to be dressed. Its edges are first, *if necessary*, gently apposed by means of isinglass or some other adhesive plaster. Either cold or warm applications may be employed. Cold or ice-water will usually be found suitable. Warm dressings—lint or soft rags soaked in warm water and covered with oiled silk, or emollient poultices—will answer better for patients who are much exhausted by previous hæmorrhage, or upon whom ligation of any considerable artery has been performed.

When there is any tendency shown by a gunshot wound towards sloughing, it is treated by charcoal poultices, by fermenting poultices, or by daily washing with a lotion containing 50 drops of nitric acid or creosote to the pint of water.

Sometimes a sinus which cannot conveniently be laid open needs to be cleansed and stimulated. This may be done by syringing with a liquid prepared like the wash just mentioned. A syringe of "hard-rubber" answers the purpose best; it should be of the capacity

---

* An instrument on this plan is described and figured in Paré's Works.

of about f℥iv, and in such order as to work well and
easily. The operator should gently introduce the pipe
of the charged instrument into one opening, some convenient vessel being placed at the other to receive the
liquid as it escapes; the body of the syringe is now to
be held perfectly steady with one hand, while with the
other the piston is pushed firmly and with some force,
but equably, forwards. Other liquids, such as astringent
solutions, and medicated washes of various kinds, are
sometimes employed in the same manner.

When a ball in its course through a limb breaks the
bone, the case becomes one of compound fracture; rules
for the dressing of these accidents will be found in
Chapter VII.

(3) *Strapping of the testicle.*—This operation is resorted to chiefly for gonorrhœal orchitis or epididymitis.
The fine hair of the part having been carefully cut away
with scissors, the surgeon provides a dozen or more
strips of adhesive plaster, about
five-eighths of an inch wide and six
or eight inches long, according to
to the degree of swelling. Having
heated and stretched one of these,
he grasps the scrotum with the
thumb and forefinger of his left
hand so as to force the testicle
down as low as possible, and then
with his right hand applies the
strip so as to keep up the pressure, its ends being crossed in
front. Several other strips suc-
ceed this, each overlapping its predecessor by about one-
fourth of an inch; their direction is changed as they

Fig. 24.

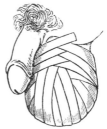

Testicle strapped with adhesive plaster.

approach the lower end of the swelling, so that the two last applied run nearly vertically from before backward. (See *Fig.* 24.) One or two strips are firmly applied around the upper part by way of confining the whole.

When in a day or two the swelling subsides, so that the cap or pouch so formed becomes loose, the strips may be sponged with spirits of turpentine to detach them, and then fresh ones be applied in the same way, the turpentine being first washed off with soap and water.

(4) *Ulcers of the legs*, when attended with varicosity of the veins, are often treated by strapping with adhesive plaster. The strips used are generally about an inch and a half in width, and eighteen or twenty inches long; they are so applied as to lie smoothly on the leg, each one overlapping its predecessor by about one-third, and the ends crossing one another in front; the successive intersections should be symmetrically arranged. As a general rule, the strapping is extended from two to four inches above and below the limits of the ulcer.

When it is desirable to make pressure over swollen joints, as in some chronic inflammatory effusions, the dressing is applied on the same principle.

CHAPTER III.

HÆMORRHAGE, whether as the result of injury or disease, or incidental to surgical operations, is a phenomenon of no trifling consequence; life itself often depends upon prompt and skilful measures for its arrest. Hence the surgeon should be familiar with the various forms it may assume, and with all the means available for checking it.

When an artery is wounded, the blood escapes in jets, synchronous with the pulsations of the heart, and is of a bright-red color. When a vein is wounded, there is a steady flow of dark purple blood. When the capillaries only are involved, there is an oozing of red blood, sometimes quite free, but not from any one point. Hence we distinguish the *arterial*, *venous* and *capillary* forms of hæmorrhage.

If, however, an artery is completely divided, the blood may flow from its distal end, (the cut extremity furthest from the heart;) it wells out very much as from a vein, unless where a free anastomosis exists, so that the impulse of a neighboring vessel is communicated to it, but its bright-red color will disclose its true source. On the other hand, a vein lying close over a large artery may, if divided, give forth its blood in jets, the throbbing of the artery being communicated to it; and here the dark color of the stream will be significant. Hence the char-

5 (45)

acters of the blood, and the mode and direction of its escape, must be taken into the account in distinguishing between arterial and venous hæmorrhage.

Secondary hæmorrhage is a most troublesome and annoying accident, which will be hereafter alluded to.

Generally speaking, the spontaneous coagulation of the blood will put a stop to its flow from wounded veins or capillaries, before any very large quantity has been lost. In some individuals, however, this tendency of the blood to coagulate seems to be wanting, and hence they are liable to profuse and dangerous bleeding from slight wounds; such a peculiarity is occasionally observed to affect whole families, and constitutes what is called the hæmorrhagic diathesis. The course of treatment to be pursued in these unfortunate cases will be hereafter detailed.

Arterial bleeding may be spontaneously arrested, by reason of four circumstances: (1) the patient becomes faint; (2) the vessel retracts itself within its sheath; (3) it contracts; (4) the blood contained in it coagulates, plugging it up. The first of these conditions acts only temporarily; the others have a permanent effect.

When a large artery, such as the femoral, is cut across, the loss of blood may be so great as to cause death by syncope, the brain being deprived of its usual stimulus and nutrition, and hence the circulation and respiration being no longer carried on. The loss of a smaller quantity of blood, as from a smaller vessel, will merely induce fainting; the heart, failing to receive its usual stimulus from the nervous system, will act but feebly, and the current of blood throughout the body will be slackened. As soon as reaction occurs, however, the activity of the circulation will be renewed, and the bleeding will be apt to recur; this is one form of second-ary hæmorrhage.

The influence of the contraction in calibre of the vessel in checking hæmorrhage is of course evident; that of its retraction is rather more complex. By this phenomenon, which is due to shortening of the obliquely-placed fibres of the outer coat of the vessel, the inner surface of the sheath is left exposed to contact with the flowing blood; this surface being irregular, the blood is entangled and coagulated upon it; moreover, the sheath itself is much more easily narrowed and closed by the pressure of the surrounding tissues than the more resist-ent artery would be.

The coagulum which forms under these circumstances is partly situated within the sheath only, but its more important portion runs up into the artery itself, obstructing its mouth, and extending in a conical shape as far up as the next branch of any size which is given off from it. Subsequently, this clot and the wall of the vessel become united, so as to constitute a dense fibrous cord.

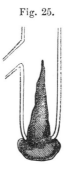

Fig. 25.

Extent of clot in a divided artery.

We have now to consider the various modes in which hæmorrhage may be arti-ficially checked; mentioning incidentally the line of treatment to be pursued in the exceptional cases already referred to, viz., those of secondary hæmorrhage, those where venous or capillary bleeding becomes excessive, and those where the hæmor-rhagic diathesis exists.

(1) *Absorbents*, such as lint, charpie, or cotton, act merely by affording a basis upon which the flowing blood

may coagulate. Agaric, a parasite of the oak, and fine dry sponge, has a like effect; and the same may be said of almost any inert powder.

(2) *Pressure* is one of the most constant resources of surgery, for the arrest or prevention of bleeding. Sometimes, in capillary hæmorrhages, it may be directly applied to the wounded surface; lint, charpie, cotton, or any available material, being spread out to the required extent, and secured until the flow of blood is stopped. Even where a small artery or arteries have been wounded, some surgeons adopt this course; but it is neither so neat nor so secure as that to be mentioned under the next head.

But where a large vessel, be it an artery or a vein, is pouring out its contents, pressure applied in this way can seldom be more than momentarily useful. Here it

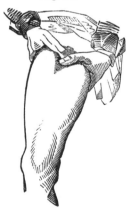

Fig. 26.

is far better to cut off the supply of blood before it reaches the wounded point; and accordingly we seek some portion of the vessel where a subjacent bone affords a firm *point d'appui* against which to compress it. Of course this pressure can only be efficient when made on the cardiac side of a wound in an artery, or the distal side of a wound in a vein.

As to the exact mode of applying the pressure, it may be done with the fingers, relieving one hand when fatigued by supporting it with the other; or the handle of a door-key, well wrapped, may be used. These expedients are, however, seldom resorted to except in cases

where the subclavian or external iliac arteries are concerned. When a wound of the scalp bleeds profusely,
the flow may be stopped by placing a thick compress on
each side of the wound, and then securing them by a
firmly-applied bandage. In like manner, on an emergency, the brachial or femoral artery may be pressed
against the subjacent bone, and so also may the radial
or ulnar. A rude appliance, but one which is invaluable in many cases of emergency, is the Spanish windlass. This is made by tying a handkerchief, rolled into

Fig. 27.

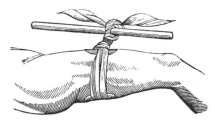

a cord, around the limb at a point above the wound; a
stick is now passed between the handkerchief and the
skin, as nearly over the artery as possible, and turned
round and round so as to twist up the handkerchief, constrict the limb, and compress the artery. (See *Fig.* 27.)
The *tourniquet*, as used in amputations, or in any operations endangering the vessels, may be employed to arrest hæmorrhage. This instrument is made after several
patterns, but the one generally supplied in amputating
cases, and most extensively used, is that devised by the
celebrated Petit, in 1718. A few circular turns of a
roller being placed around the limb, at the point where
it is desirable to compress the artery, the remainder is
brought directly over the vessel, and left there as a pad.

5*

The band of the tourniquet being now buckled over this
bandage, is tightened up to the requisite degree by turning the screw; this latter being made to bear either over
the pad, or over a point at the outer side of the limb if
the surgeon prefer it. Another plan, and a very efficient

Fig. 28.

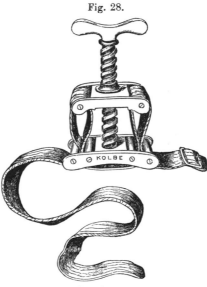

Tourniquet.

one, is to loosen that part of the strap that runs under
the body of the tourniquet, and to put into the loop thus
formed a firm roller of moderate size; now drawing the
strap tight again, placing this compress over the artery
to be controlled, buckling the strap, and turning the
screw, we have a very direct and powerful action of the
instrument secured.*   The strap of webbing, with a

---

* This plan was first suggested to me by my friend Dr. Brinton,
Surgeon U. S. V.

buckle and pad, constitutes what is called the *field tourn-*

Fig. 29.

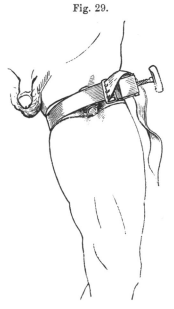

Tourniquet applied.

iquet, several of which are supplied in every army surgeon's case of instruments.

Fig. 30.

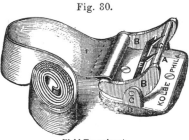

Field Tourniquet.

A tourniquet of either form above mentioned is, how-

ever, open to the objection that it constricts the whole
limb, and hence interferes with the return of venous blood.
Much ingenuity has therefore been employed in the invention of instruments for the avoidance of this difficulty. Dupuytren's compressor was one of the earliest
of these; it is very neat, but has never come into general use in this country. The "horseshoe" tourniquet,
as contrived by Signorini, and modified by Skey and
Gross, has the appearance at least of greater efficiency.

But a plan devised by the late Dr. Dorsey, of this city,
and described in his work on surgery, has the advantage
of being at once simple, reliable, and easily put in practice under almost any circumstances; it consists in placing compresses over the vessels to be controlled, and
over these a metallic band, the whole being kept in place
by a few circular turns of a roller. Wherever a patient
in danger of hæmorrhage has to be transported any considerable distance, and the more elaborate compressors
are not to be had, a knowledge of this plan may be found
of essential service.

Quite recently, the author has seen a field tourniquet
invented by Mr. Jacob Dunton, of this city, intended
for adaptation to limbs of different sizes, and for making
pressure only over the artery and the opposite point of
the circumference. It consists of two pairs of iron
plates, a strap of webbing, and a buckle. One plate of
each pair has a slit along it, in which a button-headed
screw, attached to the other, plays; their combined
length being thus regulated. The band passes through
the outer end of each plate of each pair, its upper end at
either side being caught on points at the end of the plate,
so as to fasten it as desired. A rounded block of wood
of proper size and shape, on the under surface of one

pair, serves as a pad. The modus operandi of the instrument will be readily seen.

Another method of employing pressure in the arresting of arterial hæmorrhage has been recently proposed by Dr. Simpson, of Edinburgh. It consists in inserting needles so as to pinch the vessel against the neighboring parts, close to the point at which the blood is issuing; and is called by its inventor *acupressure*, (*acus*, a needle.) As this plan has attracted a good deal of attention, I subjoin Dr. Simpson's exposition of it:—

"To produce adequate closing pressure upon any arterial tube which it is desired to constrict, the needle must be passed over it so as to compress the tube with sufficient power and force against some resisting body. Such a resisting body will be most frequently found, 1st, in the cutaneous walls and component tissues of the wound; 2d, sometimes in a neighboring bone, against which the artery may be pinned and compressed by the acupressure needle; and 3d, in a few rare cases it may possibly be found in practice that a second needle may require to be introduced to serve as a point against which the required compression is to be made. Most commonly the first of these three plans seems perfectly sufficient, and that even in amputation of the thigh. In acting upon this mode, the surgeon may place the tip of the forefinger of his left hand upon the bleeding mouth of the artery which he intends to compress and close; holding the needle in his right hand, he passes it through the *cutaneous* surface of the flap, and pushes it inwards till its point projects out to the extent of a few lines on the raw surface of the wound, a little to the right of, and anterior to his finger-tip; he then, by the action of his right hand upon the head of the needle, turns and directs the needle, so that it makes a bridge as it were *across* the site of the tube of the bleeding artery immediately in front of the point of the finger, with which he is shutting up its orifice; he next, either with this same forefinger of the left hand, or with the side of the end of the needle itself, compresses the locality of the bleeding arterial orifice and tube, and then pushes on the needle with his right hand so as to make it *re-enter* the surface of the wound a little to the left side of the artery; and, lastly, by pressing the needle further on in this direction, its point re-emerges through the *cutaneous* surface of the flap—and the site of the tube of the bleeding artery is in this way left pinned down in a compressed state by the arc or bridge of steel that is passed over it. The needle thus passes first from and through the skin of the flap *inwards* to the raw surface of the wound, and after bridging over the site of the artery, it passes secondly from the raw surface of the wound *outwards* again to and through the skin. Sometimes the needle will be best passed by the aid of the eye alone, and without guiding its course by the finger-tip applied to the bleeding orifice. It compresses not the arterial tube alone, but the structures also placed over and around the *site* of the tube. When the needle is completely adjusted, all of it that is seen on the surface of the raw wound, and that not necessarily so, is the small portion of it passing over the site of the artery, while externally, upon the cutaneous surface of the flap, we have remaining exposed more or less of its two extremities, namely, its point and its head. The rest of it is hidden in the structures of the flap or side of the wound. The degree of pressure required to close effectually the tube of an artery is certainly much less than medical practitioners generally imagine; but in the above proceeding the amount of pressure can be regulated and increased, when required, by the acuteness of the angle at which the needle is introduced and again passed out—the cutaneous and other structures of the flap serving as the resisting medium against which the needle compresses the arterial tube. But if it were ever, perchance, necessary to produce greater compression than can be thus accomplished by the needle alone, this increased pressure could be readily obtained by throwing around the two extremities of the needle exposed cutaneously a figure-of-eight ligature, as in hare-lip, with or without a small compress placed between the arc of the ligature and the skin. The process of the adjustment of the needle is difficult to describe shortly by words, but the whole of it is readily seen and imitated when repeated by a piece of cloth or leather."

This plan, although simple and ingenious, has never been very extensively employed. In some cases, it would answer extremely well; especially when the vessels to be secured were near the surface, as in amputation near the wrist.

(3) The *ligature*, now so universally known as a means of arresting the current of blood through arteries, and sometimes through veins also, was first substituted for the cautery by the great French surgeon, Paré, in 1552. Various materials have from time to time been proposed for the making of ligatures, as well as for sutures; leaden wire, cat-gut, deer-skin thongs, and silken thread. "Saddler's silk" has perhaps, however, been more employed for the purpose than anything else; it may be varied in size according to that of the vessel to be secured, but should always be round and even, and capa-

ble of withstanding a very firm pull. It should be well
waxed for use.

A ligature may be applied either to the wounded
portion of the artery, or at a point nearer the heart,

Fig. 31.   Fig. 32.

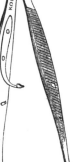

Fenestrated forceps.   Liston's forceps.

the vessel being laid bare by an incision made for the
purpose. In order to secure the end of an artery in a
wound, a hook or tenaculum may be inserted in it, or it
may be grasped with a pair of forceps; the forceps now
made are generally provided with a wedge-shaped slide,
(see *Figs.* 5 and 6,) which is pushed down through a
perforated catch attached to the other blade, so as to
ensure their hold. Some surgeons prefer the fenes-

trated forceps, (*Fig.* 31,) or the catch-forceps of Liston, (*Fig.* 32,) for this purpose. An excellent modification of the spring-forceps ordinarily supplied in the army operating-cases is shown in *Figs.* 33 and 34. It consists

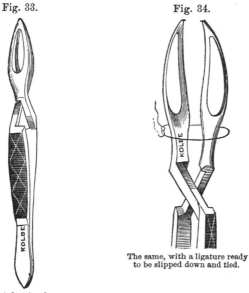

Fig. 33.

Fig. 34.

The same, with a ligature ready
to be slipped down and tied.

Fenestrated spring-forceps.

in giving them bulbous fenestrated ends, like those represented in *Fig.* 31. The advantage of this is that the ligature may be drawn tight without any risk of the knot including the tip of the instrument; the vessel, once grasped, is securely held without the hand, and there is no slide, which is always liable to rust and become useless. When from necessity or choice the surgeon is without an assistant, he may simply allow the forceps or tenaculum to hang from the end of the vessel, or he may himself hold the latter instru-

6

ment between his teeth, while his hands are engaged
in applying the ligature. Generally this duty is en-
trusted to the assistant, the operator himself picking
out the arteries with the tenaculum or forceps; the
knot should always be made on that side of the vessel
which is in view, and should be a very neat one, the
hands being changed between the loops. An ordinary
double or sailor's knot is most commonly used; the
"surgeon's knot" is made when one end of the ligature is carried twice around the other in making the first
tie. If the vessel to be secured is at the bottom of a

Fig. 35.

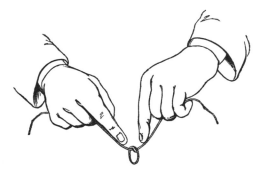

Method of tying ligature round a deeply-seated vessel.

deep wound, the operator pushes the knot down, as he
makes it, with a forefinger on each end of the thread,
rendered tense by the corresponding thumb and middle
finger. (See *Fig.* 35.) The porte-mêche described in connection with the pocket-case often answers a good purpose in thus pushing down the knot of a ligature. One
end of the ligature is cut off close, the other is allowed
to hang out at the wound. When it is necessary to

take up an artery in its continuity, it is exposed by an incision through the skin at the desired point, crossing the line of the vessel at a very acute angle; the successive layers of fascia, and the sheath of the artery, are in turn pinched up with a pair of forceps, nicked, and laid open on a grooved director; and finally the ligature is carried under the isolated vessel by means of a blunt needle with an eye near its point,* and tied as in the former case.

The immediate effect of surrounding an artery with a tightly-drawn ligature is the division of its inner and middle coats, and the occlusion of its channel; the contained blood coagulates, and sooner or later the inner coat and this coagulum become consolidated together for some distance; the clot extends as far back as the next considerable branch which is given off, just as in the case of spontaneous cessation already mentioned.

We may generally look for the separation of ligatures from the fifth to the twelfth day after that of their application; it is due to the destructive ulceration of the vessel at the strictured point. If one or more large arteries are concerned, the threads placed about them should be very carefully handled, lest they come away too soon; it is as well to leave both ends of the ligature on such a vessel, tying them together so that they may be at once recognized among the single threads securing the smaller ones.

In the dressing of wounds, it is always desirable to put a complete stop to the flow of blood, if possible;

---

* An eyed probe may answer very well in a case of emergency. If a grooved director made of silver, and therefore flexible, is at hand, it may be curved and passed under the vessel first, as a guide to the probe.

and hence the very smallest arteries which can be seen
to spring should be secured.   For this purpose a single
loop of a fine thread will suffice, and even this may be
pulled away in about twenty-four hours.

Veins are never ligatured except when divided in a
wound; the process is the same as for an artery under
like circumstances.

Torsion or twisting will sometimes close a small artery
effectively.   The vessel may be simply grasped with a
pair of forceps and twisted, or a second pair of forceps
may be applied in order to limit the twisting to a very
small extent of its length.   Mere pinching answers to
stop the bleeding from very small arteries.

(4) *Styptics*, causing not only coagulation of the flowing blood, but contraction of the wounded tissues and
their vessels, are very often indispensable.   Thus in
cases of wounds in the cavity of the upper maxillary
bone, in the vagina, rectum, fauces, etc., we often cannot
depend upon any other means; and so also when we
have to deal with a hæmorrhagic diathesis.   But to this
class of remedies there is one grave objection, viz., that
they necessarily change the surface to such an extent as
to interfere materially with the subsequent process of
healing; hence they should only be resorted to in urgent
cases.

Styptics may be used either in the solid form or in
solution; they are perhaps most efficient when powdered.
Thus finely-divided alum, sulphate of copper, or nitrate
of silver may be blown from a quill so as to reach every
portion of a wound, or either of these substances may be
used in the form of crystal, rubbed on the bleeding surface until the desired end is attained.   Strong solutions
of them may be applied with a camel's-hair pencil, or by

means of lint; the tincture of the chloride of iron, put on in the same way, is very efficient. Another article now much in vogue as a styptic is the persulphate of iron, commonly called Monsel's salt; it may be used either in substance or in strong solution, and not only causes immediate coagulation of the blood, but is in a great measure free from the caustic property so objectionable in other remedies of the kind.*

Among vegetable substances, galls, in powder or tincture, are a good deal used as hæmostatics; the powdered leaves of matico, a Peruvian plant, have also been found serviceable. Lemon-juice is sometimes employed by obstetricians in checking *post-partum* hæmorrhage, but it acts simply by exciting the uterus to contraction.

(5) *Cold* sometimes suffices of itself to check bleeding, perhaps by lowering the vital activity of the part, and also partly by causing the vessels and the tissues surrounding them to shrink. It is very readily and simply applied, cloths dipped in ice-water, or bladders filled with cold water or with pounded ice, being laid on the part. Evaporating lotions, such as diluted alcohol, may be used with a similar effect.

(6) The *actual cautery* had formerly a very much higher rank among surgical appliances than it now has; it is in fact very seldom used as a hæmostatic, on account of its formidable appearance in the eyes of the patient and his friends. It is, however, a very efficient, and by no means a very painful resource. At all events, when

---

* Dr. Pancoast, of Philadelphia, is in the habit of using a styptic composed as follows: Carbonate of potash ʒj, Castile soap ʒij, alcohol fℨiv. Although intensely painful when applied, this preparation is extremely efficient, and can almost always be readily obtained. Its mode of action is difficult to explain.

we are desirous of checking hæmorrhage promptly, and
other means are either unattainable or unavailing, this
may and ought to be brought into service. The iron
should not be heated beyond blackness, and should be
thoroughly applied to every point of the wound which is
giving forth blood. Its shape does not matter much,
provided it is large enough to act over some extent of
surface, and small enough to be carried completely into
any portion of the wound; but if the surgeon provides
himself with only one, that one ought to be of a wedge
or hatchet-shape, as combining the greatest range of applications. When several irons are kept, they may all
be adapted to a single wooden handle, and shifted as the
occasion demands.

It may be well, in conclusion, to sum up the relative
values of the different means of arresting hæmorrhage
which have now been described.

During an operation, or for any temporary purpose,
we prevent bleeding by the use of the tourniquet, or by
pressure applied in any convenient way to the arterial
trunk going to the part. Venous hæmorrhage need not
generally be interfered with except in very old or young
patients, or in those who are very feeble; ligation or
pressure should be used to check it in such cases.
Arterial bleeding will be best arrested permanently by
ligation, or by acupressure, as proposed by Simpson, in
cases where this can be effectively used. General oozing
from a surface may be combated by pressure directly
applied, by ice held to the part, by styptics, or in some
rare instances by the actual cautery.

SUTURES.

SUTURES are very valuable when the parts to be held in apposition are composed of lax and yielding tissue, or are of such a form that no purchase is afforded for adhesive strips or other means; on account also of the accuracy with which a wound may be closed by them, they are much used in injuries of the face, where it is of course very desirable to avoid scars. Their employment has been strongly opposed by some writers on surgery, but is quite in vogue at the present day.

Various materials are or have been used for making sutures. "Saddler's silk" answers very well; other animal substances, such as deer-sinews, catgut, and buckskin rolled into slender thongs, have also been employed, although not to any very great extent. Upon an emergency, very fine linen twine might be of service. But metallic wire, gold, silver, iron or lead, bids fair to supersede all other articles for this purpose, having been brought into notice mainly by Dr. J. Marion Sims, of New York, to whom surgery is much indebted for his earnest advocacy of this long-neglected idea. Iron-wire for sutures has been placed on the army supply-table.

Flat needles, more or less curved, are used for passing the thread or wire; they should be double-edged from the point to the widest part, and large enough to prevent any dragging of the skin as the suture is drawn through. The shapes generally used are shown in *Fig.* 36. If thread is used, the ends are tied together in a smooth double knot, or in very rare instances knotted separately; if wire, the ends are first crossed so as to make a single knot, and then twisted upon one another; in either case they are cut off close.

When the tissues involved are lax and yielding, as in the eyelid, the suture may be passed close to the edges

Fig. 36.

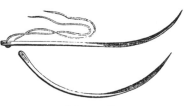

Suture needles.

of the wound; if they are firmer and more resisting, a stronger hold must be secured. Care must be taken never to include more than the skin and subjacent areolar tissue.

Several different forms of suture are employed: the interrupted, the twisted or hare-lip, the continued, the quilled, the dry, and the button. These have now to be successively considered.

(1) The *interrupted* suture consists of separate loops

Fig. 37.

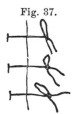

Interrupted suture.

or *points*, placed at greater or less intervals according to the size of the wound, the shape of its edges, and its greater or less tendency to gape; much judgment may be shown in their distribution. Any irregularities in the line of the wound are advantageous, since they serve as guides for that exact coaptation of the edges which is essential to prevent subsequent deformity; the rule is always to secure first the flap, (the largest if there be several,) or the middle of each lip if the wound be straight.

Either one or two needles may be used in making the interrupted suture. In the former case, the skin is pierced at one side of the wound from without inwards, at the other from within outwards; in the latter, both needles are passed from within outwards. I have always noticed, however, that patients complain most when the skin is penetrated from within; so that it seems to me better to follow the first-named plan. Some surgeons use the same needle twice, carrying it from within outwards with each end of the thread, but there does not seem to be any advantage in so doing.

Adhesive strips are generally applied in the interspaces between the sutures, so as to prevent the latter from being too much drawn upon by the surrounding tissues.

Generally speaking, sutures accomplish their object in two or three days; and hence they need be no longer kept in place. They should be removed earlier, if rendered tense by the swelling of the part; sometimes this may be foreseen, and the loops loosely fastened in the first instance. In order to remove a point of the interrupted suture, raise the knot a little with a pair of forceps, pass one blade of a pair of scissors beneath the thread or wire, so as to cut it without any jerk, and then draw it out by the knot.

(2) The *twisted* suture is a modification of the foregoing; it is made by passing a pin through both edges of the wound to be closed, and drawing them together upon it by means of a waxed thread applied in the form of a figure-of-8. Being chiefly employed in operations for the deformity known as hare-lip, this suture is called the *hare-lip* suture, and the pins *hare-lip* pins. The pins may be made of steel, or of silver; it has been proposed to make them of silver, with steel points which may be removed when their introduction has been effected.

But any sort of wire answers the purpose; a common needle is as good as anything else.

Fig. 38.

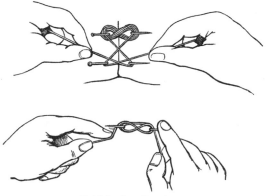

Twisted or hare-lip suture.

In most cases, two or more pins have to be inserted; this may be done either with a pair of forceps, (the small forceps of every pocket-case being grooved in each blade so as to take a firm hold of the head of an ordinary hare-lip pin,) or by means of the fingers alone. All the pins may be first introduced, and the ligature then applied, if a careful assistant is at hand to support the edges of the wound; otherwise it is better to secure each one as it is inserted. The loops of each figure-of-8 go, as a matter of course, behind the pin, then crossing in front, just over the wound; the former should be made to spread out over the skin, so as to press upon a somewhat extensive surface. The points of the pins should be either cut off or covered with wax, lest they should injure the skin.

After about forty-eight hours have elapsed the pins may be withdrawn, by grasping them with a pair of forceps, and pulling upon them gently with a slight rotatory motion; the thread may be left until it becomes loose of itself. I have elsewhere mentioned (Chap. II., p. 36) a modification of the hare-lip suture which I have found very useful in incised wounds, the pins being passed parallel to the cut edges, and their free ends drawn towards one another by means of thread or wire.

Another form of suture, acting on the same principle as that just described, is employed by some surgeons. Instead of the figure-of-8 turns of thread or wire, small loops of India-rubber are cast over the free ends of each needle; they may be very easily made by cutting thin transverse sections of a fine gum-elastic tube. I have chiefly seen this plan employed by my friend Dr. W. L. Atlee, after the operation of ovariotomy, but do not know whether it was original with him.

(3) The *continued* suture is very little used, except in sewing up bodies after post-mortem examinations. It is begun at one end of the wound, by carrying the thread from without inwards, across, and through the other lip from within outwards; the loop so inserted is tied, and the thread is then carried from one lip to the other, always passing from within outwards, until at the other extremity of the wound it is closed off by tying, just as at the starting-point.

The objections to this form of suture are, that its track is very extensive, and therefore slow to heal, and that it puckers up the edges of the wound more than any other suture does.

(4) The *quilled* suture has fallen rather undeservedly

into disuse; its great merit is the uniform pressure made by it along the edges of the wound. It is made by carrying a suitable number of double ligatures (a loop of the thread being passed through the eye of the needle) through both lips of the wound; a quill, a small roll of lint, or a piece of gum-elastic bougie is now passed through the loops on one side, and another is placed between the double row of ends on the other; now by tying these ends as firmly as may be required, we evidently bring the quills together, and thus press the edges of the wound against one another.

(5) The *dry* suture is very seldom employed; it is made by applying a strip of adhesive plaster parallel with each margin of the wound, and then sewing these strips together by their adjacent edges.

(6) The *button* suture is one which has recently been brought into very great repute by the success obtained by means of it in cases of vesico-vaginal fistula. Much use might also be made of it in operations for cleft palate, and perhaps in some cases of unnatural anus. For detailed descriptions of the various forms of this suture, the reader is referred to the writings of Sims, Bozeman, Simpson, and Brown. Suffice it to say here, that the principle involved is the securing of the suture, which is almost invariably metallic, by clamping it over a metallic shield fitted to the surface of the closed wound or fissure.

CHAPTER IV.

DEPLETION by surgical means may be practised upon the system at large, when it is said to be *general*, or upon a special organ or organs, when it is said to be *local*. The former has been to a great extent abandoned at the present day, although it was long looked upon as indispensable in the treatment of every inflammatory complaint. The latter is still, and probably always will be, an important resource. Both are called for sufficiently often to make it necessary for the practitioner to know how to employ them himself, in case he should be unable to procure the services of a person who makes it his business to do so.

General depletion is most frequently performed by the opening of a vein, called also *venesection* or *phlebotomy*. The operation consists in obstructing the flow of blood towards the heart so as to render the vein turgid, opening the vein, letting out as much blood as may be desired, and closing the little wound. One of the veins near the bend of the arm is generally chosen, bleeding from the jugular and the saphena being almost entirely abandoned at present: horses are often bled from the ranine vein, under the tongue, and it has been proposed to open this vein for the relief of angina, tonsillitis, etc. in the human subject.

For the ordinary operation of bleeding from the arm,

7 (69)

we require simply a sharp lancet, two strips of bandage, a compress of lint, and a vessel of some kind to receive the blood as it flows.* Water and towels are of course necessary for the subsequent cleansing of the part.

There are two kinds of lancet in use.

The THUMB-LANCET consists of a rather broad blade, an inch and a half or two inches in length, double-edged where it tapers towards its point. Its handle is formed of two thin plates of tortoise shell, a little longer and wider than the blade, and fastened together as well as to it by means of a pivot. Very little importance attaches to the exact shape of the blade, but it should always be in perfect order, as sharp as possible, and kept scrupulously clean.

The SPRING-LANCET consists of a blade or fleam set in a small case, and driven down by a spring when a trigger or button is pressed upon. It is so contrived that the distance to which it flies can be regulated to suit the greater or less size or depth of the vein to be operated upon. Authorities are somewhat at variance as to the relative advantages of this instrument and the thumb-lancet, but a skilful operator need hardly hesitate to choose between the two; the thumb-lancet is, however, a more surgical weapon, and from its simplicity is more easily kept in order.

When this last-named instrument is used, a strip of bandage is first tied round the arm, tightly enough to

---

* If the operator is a young surgeon acting under directions, or if he desires to record the exact amount of blood taken, it will be well for him to use a graduated bowl, such as may be obtained at any apothecary shop.

cause turgidity of the veins. The surgeon then opens his lancet so that the blade and handle are at right angles, and lays it in any convenient place, or according to some teachers takes it in his mouth, carefully keeping the point away from the hand with which he intends to operate. His position should be on the inner side of the right arm, on the outer side of the left, if he be right-handed, and *vice versâ*. Now, controlling the flow through the vein with one thumb, lest the blood should spirt too forcibly at first, he takes the blade of the lancet between the other thumb and forefinger, and rests the little finger of this hand upon the forearm, so that the point of the lancet blade is just over the swollen vein. By the straightening out of the thumb and forefinger, the point is now carried down into the vein, across it, and out again through the skin, describing an arc of a circle. The line of incision should be at an acute angle with the axis of the vessel. Of course the wall of the vein is simply nicked, and not divided in its whole circumference. Some care is requisite in order that the skin and the wall of the vein be cut at corresponding points; the skin should be slightly stretched by grasping the member with the hand not holding the lancet. When the incision is properly made, a continuous jet of blood issues from the orifice, and is received into the vessel provided for the purpose.

When a vein is opened by a large incision, the quantity of blood lost in a given time will be greater than that which would escape through a small orifice. If the patient sits up during the operation, he will faint sooner than if he were lying down. Hence if we wish to produce syncope, we let the patient sit up, and make a free incision; if we wish to abstract a good deal of blood,

without much immediate effect, we cause him to lie down,
and let the blood flow slowly.

Should the flow of blood be sluggish, or should it cease,
the patient should be made to work his fingers, or to
grasp any convenient object; or friction of the skin along
the course of the vein may be resorted to.   A sufficient
quantity having been taken, the
constricting band may be removed, and the compress placed
firmly upon the wound and held
there; the flow being thus checked, the limb is cleansed of any
blood with which it may have become soiled, and dried, when the
compress is bound in place by
means of a clean strip of bandage.

When the spring-lancet is employed, the procedure is exactly
the same as that now described,
except of course that the operating hand is held perfectly still,
the fleam alone moving, and one
finger only being used to touch
the trigger or button.

Almost every one must be familiar with the appearance of the
swollen veins of the bend of the
arm; but the annexed cut will
show the normal anatomy of the
part.   Generally the median cephalic (h) or median basilic (g) is
selected for opening.

Certain accidents are liable to

Fig. 39.

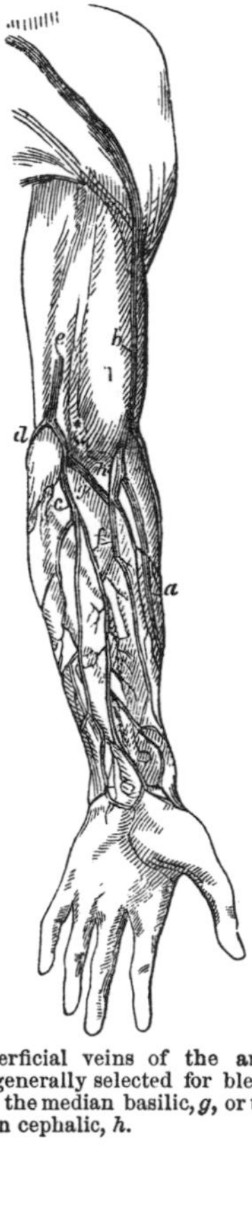

Superficial veins of the arm.
That generally selected for bleeding is the median basilic, g, or the
median cephalic, h.

happen either at the time of bleeding, or subsequently; they are mostly of trifling consequence, but it is as well that the surgeon should know of them beforehand.

(1) *Ecchymosis* may occur from a slight want of parallelism between the wound in the vein and that in the skin. It is of no moment, and will disappear of itself in a few days.

(2) *Thrombus* is a more pronounced degree of ecchymosis, the effused blood constituting a clot in the areolar tissue. Very rarely, such a clot may act as a foreign body, and excite suppuration; generally it is soon and easily absorbed. Should the local action, however, be more troublesome, the arm ought to be placed at rest on a splint, and soothing applications made to it.

(3) A small cutaneous nerve may be wounded. This will be apt to cause pain, but no other bad effect.

(4) The artery may be wounded through the vein; an occurrence manifested by the escape of florid blood in jets Pressure over the vein below the opening does not arrest this jetting stream, but compression of the brachial artery against the humerus does control it. (In case of a high bifurcation of the brachial, it would be necessary to press upon the axillary; and this should be done if the bleeding is *not* stopped by compressing the brachial, in order to remove all doubt.) We have to dread, from this accident, the formation of a false aneurism, setting up a communication between the artery and vein, or the persistence of a mere orifice between the two vessels. Velpeau recommends in these cases the immediate application of a compress, graduated so as to bear upon the point of lesion, and held in place by a firm bandage; this dressing to be retained for from five to fifteen days. Should this fail, ligation of the artery would become necessary.

7*

(5) A vein in which bleeding has been practised may become inflamed, either from the lancet used or the dressing having been charged with some irritating matter, or from an unhealthy state of the patient's system. An unfavorable result is very apt to ensue in such cases, unless when the irritation is merely local; rest and soothing applications, with cleanliness, are then generally sufficient to allay it. In other cases the treatment must be more active; the reader is referred to works on general surgery for its details. Erythema may attack these wounds, like any other, and is treated in the same way.

(6) It occasionally happens that a small lymphatic vessel is wounded, and takes on inflammatory action; the same remarks apply to this case as to that of phlebitis.

(7) *Syncope* or fainting is very apt to occur, in timid patients, from the mere sight of the flowing blood; the stream should then be checked at once, at least until the head is lowered, and the system has had time to react fully. Should any considerable amount of blood have been already lost, the fainting may be looked upon as an indication that the operation ought to be stopped.

(8) Some writers have attached importance to the wounding of the tendon of the biceps in venesection; but it is really a matter of no moment.

Bleeding in the hand is easily performed, by allowing the part to hang down, at the same time compressing the lower portion of the arm, and when the veins have become turgid, opening the largest one which presents itself at the back of the metacarpal bone of the thumb. The operation is conducted in exactly the same way as in the forearm.

A vein may be opened in the foot, much in the same

manner. It is customary to place the foot in warm
water, to promote the flow of blood, and even to keep it
immersed until a sufficient effect has been produced.
This operation is very seldom, if ever, employed in this
country; it presents no special advantages.

Bleeding from the external jugular vein was at one
time much practised in cases of cerebral disease or injury, with a view of unloading the vessels of the head.
But there is no special advantage in opening this vein;
it is less easily operated upon than other veins, and there
is more danger of the entrance of air into it, so as to
cause death by distension of the heart.   The operation,
if considered desirable in any case, is performed on pre-
cisely the same principles as that practised on the arm.
Pressure is made upon the vein so as to engorge it, by
means of a compress placed just above the clavicle, and
kept firm by a cravat or bandage passing across to the
opposite axilla; the incision is effected as low down at
least as the middle portion of the vessel, and generally
a little lower.   As a general rule, it is necessary to
use a little trough of paper or card-board to guide the
stream of blood, and prevent its trickling down over the
skin.

The danger of the entrance of air into the vein,
already mentioned, may be to a great extent obviated by
closing the wound before the compress is removed from
above the clavicle.   But in fact this operation is now
little practised, except in cases of emergency, as in
threatened apoplexy, or in some forms of infantile con-
vulsions.

ARTERIOTOMY is at the present day almost entirely
abandoned.   It is practised only upon the temporal

artery or its anterior branch, and that in extremely rare instances. A sharp-pointed, curved bistoury may be inserted beneath the vessel, and made to cut its way out, or a scalpel may be used to cut first the skin and then the artery. In either case the section of the vessel should be complete. Generally the blood spirts out in jets, but sometimes a little trough of card-board or tin may be required to lead the blood away from the skin.

When enough blood has escaped, a compress and firm bandage are applied, just as in cases of accidental hæmorrhage. The only subsequent danger is that of the formation of an aneurism, but it is very trifling.

LOCAL DEPLETION is performed by scarifications, leeches or cups. In all these methods, the same principle is involved, the pressure of the atmosphere causing the blood to flow through openings in the minuter ramifications of the vascular system.

(1) *Scarification.*—This may often be performed simply by making a number of incisions, of no great depth or length, in the inflamed part; a lancet, scalpel or bistoury answering equally well for the purpose. Less pain is caused, however, by the use of the instrument known as a *scarificator*, which consists of a number of blades set in a frame, and worked by a trigger, the extent of their protrusion, and therefore the depth of the wound, being regulated by means of a screw; sixteen or twenty incisions are thus effected simultaneously. Bleeding may be encouraged, if necessary, by a poultice or a warm water-dressing.

Scarification with a lancet or bistoury is sometimes resorted to for the relief of œdema; it is so simple an operation as to require no special description here.

Sometimes the mucous membrane about the upper part of the larynx becomes œdematous, so as to threaten suffocation; it then has to be scarified, by means of a very sharp gum-lancet. Where other portions of the mucous membrane of the mouth or fauces require to be incised, a gum-lancet or a bistoury may be employed at the convenience of the operator.

(2) *Cupping.*—This operation receives its name from the small glasses shaped like a bell or cup, which are used in performing it. As kept in the shops, these glasses are generally in sets, with a small exhausting pump which fits a pipe on the top of each cup. Applying the margin of a cup to the skin, the air may be pumped out through the tube, and the atmospheric pressure on the parts around will cause the portion of skin covered by the cup to swell up into it, becoming red and turgid. There is a stop-cock on each tube, by closing which the cup may be left adhering to the surface. Another way of rarefying the air, when the pump is not available, is by burning a little bit of paper in the glass; the air is thus not only heated, but deprived of its oxygen, and the cup may be quickly inverted and applied with a satisfactory effect. Cups are removed by simply turning the stop-cock and allowing the air to rush in; and when the plain glass ones are used, by inserting the finger-nail under the edge, so as to raise it slightly and admit the air. The process now described is called *dry* cupping; we say that so many *dry cups* have been applied to a part.

Cut cups are said to be used, when the swollen area of skin is incised either with a lancet or scarificator; the latter instrument is the one generally employed. It is necessary, in order to take away blood to any extent at all, to reapply the cup after the cutting has been accomplished; and this may be done as often as seems desirable. About an ounce is generally drawn by each cup, but the amount will vary somewhat, according to the vascularity of the part, the size of the glasses used, the state of the blood, etc. It is not very often necessary to apply any dressing after cupping, but if the skin is tender it may be protected by a piece of lint spread with cerate, or by a water-dressing, warm or cold according to the feelings of the patient.

Cups should never be applied directly to an inflamed portion of skin, but in the neighborhood of it; they are very useful as a means of counter-irritation when put on over congested or inflamed viscera. They should not be applied in cases where there is much emaciation, or over bones which are but thinly covered. Some parts, as for instance the eyelids, are too small or of too lax texture to allow of the application of ordinary cups to them; but it has been proposed to substitute smaller ones in such cases. This idea originated in France, as did also that of exhausting or rarefying the air around entire limbs, first brought forward by M. Junod. For the latter purpose a cylinder is used, of sufficient size, having a caoutchouc band around the extremity at which the limb enters, which adapts itself to the surface of the latter so as to exclude the air. The contained air is pumped out, the degree of rarefaction being measured by an arrangement called a *manomètre*. Jamain speaks of this process as powerfully revulsive.

The application of cups, or at least of an instrument acting on the same principle, to the interior surface of the uterus, has been proposed by Dr. Storer, of Boston.* He ascribes the conception of the idea to Prof. Simpson, of Edinburgh, and seems strongly impressed with its value in some cases of defective menstruation.

Mention should here be made of an instrument called the *bdellomètre*, invented by M. Sarlandière; it is merely a combination of the cupping-glass and the scarificator, the latter being worked by a stem passing through the top of the former. Its expensiveness and complexity, and the difficulty of keeping it in order, will always prevent this instrument from being very widely used.

(3) *Leeches.*—These animals have from a very early period been employed for the remedial abstraction of blood. They are sometimes obtained from brooks, but more generally from stagnant water; their efficiency varies with their size, freshness, and state of health.

Leeches are divided, medically speaking, into the American and the Swedish; although they are imported not only from Sweden, but also from Poland, Bohemia, and Turkey. The back is in both varieties of a very dark-green color, almost black, but the American leech has a reddish-brown belly, while that of the European is greenish-yellow, with two rows of black spots. But the important difference between them lies in the unequal amounts of blood which they will draw. An American leech may be expected to abstract somewhat over a fluidrachm, half a dozen being put on by a leecher for every ounce of blood he is desired to take. The imported leech is of larger capacity, and its bite bleeds more freely afterwards than that of the American does; the patient losing in all rather more than half an ounce for each one.

---

* Am. Journ. of the Med. Sciences, Jan., 1858.

Leeches draw blood by suction upon the triangular wound which they make in biting; their jaws are three in number, cartilaginous, and provided each with two rows of fine teeth, about sixty in each row. Those of medium size will generally bite best; their skins are glossy, and their movements powerful and active, if they are in good condition.

If the part to which leeches are to be applied is at all hairy, it should be shaved; both because they will take hold better, and because the hair would otherwise become matted with blood. If the leeches do not bite readily, the skin may be rubbed, so as to bring the blood to its superficial vessels; or a little warm milk and water, or sweetened water, may be applied to it. Another plan is to obtain a drop of blood, by squeezing the finger so as to congest its tip, which is then punctured; and to moisten the surface with this. When the application is to be made within a certain area, the leeches may be placed within a glass vessel of suitable size, which is then inverted over the part; a towel may be used in the same way, and will answer better if a larger space is to be embraced. Another plan is to apply the leeches one by one, placing each in a glass tube, the buccal extremity of the animal towards the surface it is to attack; the end of the tube being placed upon this surface, the leech may be pushed toward it, and will generally bite at once. This plan is especially useful for the mucous membranes, for obvious reasons; but it has the disadvantage of giving rather more pain than when all the leeches take hold at the same time. A roll of paper answers very well instead of the glass tube, when this latter is not to be had; if the application is to be made within the rectum or vagina, the passage should be dilated with a suitable speculum before the tube is introduced.

When leeches are full of blood, they generally drop off from their hold. If they do not, they may be made to let go by putting a little salt or snuff upon their backs; but they should never be pulled upon, lest their teeth be detached and remain in the wound.

Several methods have been proposed for making each leech draw more blood than he naturally would—such for instance as cutting off the caudal extremity of the animal. This plan is not only cruel, but it often causes leeches to drop off at once, and must of course render them useless for any subsequent application.

After leeches have let go, or have been removed, the flow of blood is apt still to continue. When it is desirable that this flow should take place, it may be encouraged by a warm water-dressing, a poultice, or even by the application of a cupping-glass. Occasionally, however, it is necessary to stop the bleeding instead of promoting it; and this may be done in various ways. Cold water, cold astringent lotions—solution of alum, or of sulphate of zinc or copper, ℥ss to the ounce—a pointed stick of nitrate of silver inserted into each bite, dusting the surface with any astringent powder, or the application of a finely pointed cauterizing iron at a black heat, may be tried. The muriated tincture of iron, or a solution of the persulphate of iron, (Monsel's salt,) may succeed when other means fail. Bourgery states that Richerand saw the temporal artery, and Dupuytren the external jugular vein, wounded by leech-bites. Larrey saw several soldiers who had alarming hæmatemesis after swallowing some leeches in drinking water; in such cases any mild emetic, or a dose of salt and water, would be administered with propriety, and would probably cause the ejection of the worms. A wound of a superficial artery or vein would require compression, and if this failed, the ligature.

Enough blood having been taken, and the flow having ceased, a little lint spread with cerate may be applied as a dressing if any be required; very often it suffices simply to protect the part by laying over it a piece of soft linen rag. As a permanent scar is always left by the bite of leeches, they should not be unnecessarily applied to parts where such a scar would be unsightly, especially in females.

Before this subject is dismissed, a few remarks must be made in reference to the keeping of leeches. They thrive best in river-water, in which a few aquatic plants are growing; and the vessel containing them should be protected from the direct rays of the sun. Some mud and gravel should form the bottom of the tank, and the water should not be often renewed, lest the very delicate young leeches should be washed away and lost. After being used, leeches should be kept for six or seven months in a reservoir of clay or earth; this is better than to make them disgorge the blood by squeezing, or by putting them in salt water. Some think that they should never be employed more than once; and they certainly should not, if the patient from whom they have drawn blood has had any specific disorder.

Mechanical Leeches.—These are small tubes, which are sold in sets like cupping-glasses, with a pump for exhausting the air, and a lancet for scarifying the skin. Where real leeches cannot be obtained, these answer a very good purpose.

M. Lüer, the well-known instrument-maker of Paris,

supplies an excellent form of mechanical leech. It consists of a strong glass tube, three or four inches in length, open at one end, the edge of which is ground smooth, and furnished at the other with an ebony stopper; through the centre of this stopper plays freely a screw, terminating in a cork which fits tightly in the tube. A nut on the screw draws it up through the stopper, and thus raises the cork, so as to make strong suction upon the skin to which the open end of the tube is applied. In order to open the cutaneous vessels, a very simple instrument is used. A short and wide brass tube, perforated with two holes at the side, has within it another, around which two or three turns of a string are taken, the end of the string passing through the holes in the outside tube. Running through the inside tube is a steel bar, terminating in a tube of small calibre, whose free end is ground into a circular cutting edge; the bar is fixed, by a screw passing through the wall of the second tube, so as to *set* the circular knife to any depth desired. Now by pressing the knife against the skin, and pulling quickly upon the ends of the string alternately, a circular cut is made, over which the glass tube is placed, and suction made by drawing up the cork, which acts as a piston.

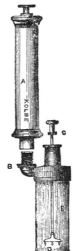

Fig. 40.

Kolbè's mechanical leech.

Mr. Kolbè, of Philadelphia, furnishes an artificial leech such as is shown in *Fig.* 40. E is the suction-tube applied to the skin, the punctures being made by means of the points at D, the rod C playing air-tight in the cap of the suction-tube. A pump, A, screwing on at B to a branch of the tube, E, serves to exhaust the air in the latter, and thus to draw the blood from the punctures made in the skin, just as the natural leech would do by means of its sucker.

CHAPTER V.

MANY surgical procedures are greatly facilitated by placing the patient or the part to be dealt with in a state of insensibility. The surgeon is unembarrassed by cries, complaints or struggles. The patient escapes not only the pain, but the recollection of it, which to a nervous person is nearly as bad, and is moreover saved the necessity of a fearful effort, successful or otherwise, at self-control.

Anæsthesia is said to be *general* or *local*, according as it is made to affect the entire system of the patient, or only the part to be examined or operated upon.

1. GENERAL ANÆSTHESIA.—All the narcotics, opium, belladonna,.etc., have the power of dulling pain; but they not only fail to completely overcome it, but their action is so slow, so prolonged, and in many respects so hurtful, that they are used only as palliatives and auxiliaries.

Alcoholic intoxication renders its subject insensible to pain, but there are obvious objections to its intentional production for this purpose, aside from its uncertainty and its danger.

Sulphuric ether and *chloroform*, in the form of vapors administered by inhalation, have superseded almost entirely all other general anæsthetics. The former, which

8*　　　　(85)

is the agent chiefly employed in this country, is obtained by the action of sulphuric acid on alcohol; it is
in fact merely a dehydrated alcohol. Its effects, when
inhaled, are first exhilaration, then violent excitement,
and finally complete insensibility. About f℥viij are
generally required for an adult, but some persons are
more susceptible to it than others, and much more will of
course be given if the anæsthesia is kept up for a length
of time. Nausea, and vomiting of whatever may be in
the stomach, are usually observed as the patient comes
to. Consciousness is soon recovered, but there is for
several hours a state of more or less mental confusion,
and an odor of ether may be perceived in the breath for
several days. Altogether, the symptoms are much like
those of alcoholic intoxication, but are less lasting, and
pass in quicker succession. Nor is there so great a degree of ensuing depression; headache also is infrequent
after the inhalation of ether. No case of death from the
moderate employment of ether is on record.* Its inflam-
mability should be borne in mind when it is administered
anywhere near a candle or gas-light.

Chloroform is preferred by some surgeons of eminence
in the United States, and by many abroad, to ether.
It is obtained by the distillation of chloride of lime with
rectified spirit. Its effects are a good deal like those of
ether, but a much smaller quantity, f℥j to f℥ij, is needed
to produce them. It is pleasanter than ether, but more
dangerous, many cases of death from its use having
occurred.

Neither of these agents should be administered to any

---

* The habitual use of ether, however, induces symptoms and
pathological changes closely analogous to those of alcoholism.

one laboring under serious organic disease of the brain, heart or lungs, especially the two former. After some of the deaths from chloroform, however, it does not appear that there was found any adequate cause of this kind to account for the fatal result.

From what has been said, it may be seen that a much greater degree of risk and responsibility is involved in giving chloroform than in giving ether. If the surgeon decides upon taking that risk, he should in the first place be sure that the article to be used is of the best quality. He should secure the services of a competent and careful assistant to watch the pulse and respiration.* The chloroform should be poured into a hollow cone formed of a new stiff towel, the base of which should then be placed over the mouth and nose of the patient. If the upper end of the cone be closed, care should be taken to suspend the inhalation for a second or two every few minutes, so that some air may enter the lungs along with the vapor. Prof. Simpson of Edinburgh has lately described another method of administering chloroform, which I have found to answer extremely well for either this article or ether. This is to lay over the patient's face a thin rag or handkerchief, upon which, at the part corresponding to the mouth and nose, the anæsthetic is allowed to fall drop by drop, until the desired effect is produced. Less chloroform is used in this way, while

---

* Chloroform has been found much more available for field use, by our army surgeons, than ether; being more portable and convenient, as well as more prompt in its effects. It was most successfully employed also in the Crimea, both by the English and French surgeons; although the former bear stronger testimony to its merits than the latter.

the process is easier, quicker, and in the opinion of some safer, than the method usually adopted.

The curious fact has been noted, that chloroform acts more speedily when administered in the open air.

The cone should be instantly removed upon any marked change being noticed in the pulse, the breathing, or the pupils. Should the patient sink, cold affusion, stimulation to the surface, and artificial respiration should instantly be resorted to, the tongue being drawn forward with a tenaculum.

Sulphuric ether is usually poured into the hollow of a cone-shaped sponge, previously wrung out of water. To prevent waste by evaporation, a towel, or by some practitioners a tin cap, is placed over the sponge. According to Dr. Lente,* of Cold Spring, N. Y., it is desirable to have as little air as possible mixed with the inhaled ether; and this idea has certainly been justified by the results of my experience. My own practice is, when I do not employ Simpson's plan, already described, to stand behind the patient's head, grasping it between my open hands, and steadying the sponge, applied over the nose and mouth, between my thumbs; thus, after the first gradual approach of the sponge, making it next to impossible for the patient to get his face away from it, and at the same time avoiding all risk of squeezing the sponge and wasting the ether. At the same time I keep urging the patient to blow through the sponge, in order to obtain the succeeding deep inspiration. Complete etherization is indicated by total loss of voluntary motion, and absence of pain when the conjunctiva is

---

* New York Journal of Medicine, Sept., 1855, and American Journal of the Med. Sciences, April, 1861, p. 357.

touched. It may be kept up safely so long as the breathing is not stertorous; or the sponge may be withdrawn, and reapplied if necessary.

Amylene, a very volatile and fetid substance, was proposed a few years ago as an anæsthetic by M. Giraldés of Paris and M. Caillot of Strasbourg; but its disagreeable properties, and the fact that a patient to whom it was administered by Dr. Snow of London died from its effects, have caused it to be laid aside.

Kerosolene, a liquid hydro-carbon obtained by the distillation of coal, has been lately brought forward in Boston as an anæsthetic. It is said to be effectual, tasteless, with an unirritating vapor, and is cheap. Its value has not yet been sufficiently tested.

2. LOCAL ANÆSTHESIA.—This may be produced in very various ways. We have not here to speak of anodyne liniments, poultices or fomentations, for the relief of existing pain, but only of the prevention of suffering from surgical procedures.

Cold has been successfully employed to render painless the removal of the toe-nail, of superficial tumors, etc.; but it does not answer when the deeper-seated tissues must be attacked. It is applied by means of the ordinary freezing mixture of pounded ice and salt. A sufficient quantity of this is wrapped in a piece of lint or rag, and laid over the part, which in a few minutes loses its color and temperature, and becomes hard; it may now be cut without causing any pain.

Electricity has been used in some cases to advantage, especially in the extraction of teeth. It is however somewhat uncertain, and is apt itself to give rise to disagreeable or even painful sensations. The mode of ap-

plying it is generally by connecting one pole from a
battery with the instrument to be used, and the other
with the patient's hand by an ordinary handle or re-
ophore.   As yet, this means has not been developed to
any degree of importance; and in view of its uncertainty
and the momentary duration of its action, we may doubt
whether it ever will be.

CHAPTER VI.

BANDAGES.

The material commonly used for bandages is muslin, of medium thickness. If too heavy, it will not adapt itself readily enough to the shape of the part; if too light, it will yield too much. Washing deprives it of its elasticity, and therefore renders it less useful for most surgical purposes.

Linen is much less elastic than muslin, and much more expensive; it is therefore seldom used. Flannel is employed when we want warmth, elasticity and softness; but it must be remembered that if the patient should perspire, the bandage may become too tight when it dries again, as this material shrinks under such circumstances.

The form of bandage most extensively employed is the roller; a strip of muslin, from two to three inches wide and from five to ten yards long, according to the part to be bound up, being rolled up into a cylinder for use. Each roller should consist of only one strip; when two or more pieces are sewed together, the seams cause welts and excoriations if the bandage is applied with any degree of tightness. The selvedges should be carefully torn off from the piece of muslin used for bandages, for the same reason. For obvious reasons, the warp of the stuff should be exactly followed, lest the strips be crooked; it is therefore better to tear bandages off than to cut them.

Bandages may be rolled up for use, either with a machine or by hand. The machine employed is very simple, the end of the strip being placed on a metal pin, which is turned by a crank; the ends of the pin rest in two uprights, fixed in a board, which for greater

Fig. 41.

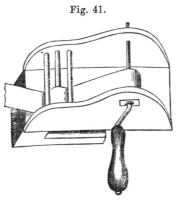

Bandage-roller.

steadiness may be screwed to a table. A guide may be obtained either by an upright board with one or more slits in it, or by two or more round cross-bars between the uprights. When the strip is rolled up, the pin and crank may be disengaged, and the roller slipped off from the pin. Much labor is saved by a contrivance of this kind, when many bandages are to be rolled.

But the surgeon is very often so placed, that he must dispense with any such aid; and then a knowledge of the proper mode of rolling bandages by hand is indispensable. The process is very simple, and a little practice will make it very easy.

One end of the strip is doubled over for about eight inches, and laid on the thigh, the foot resting on a chair or other support; the surgeon then folds the doubled part on itself. Again and again this folding is repeated, until a body is formed around which can be rolled the adjoining part of the strip. This rolling is done between the hand and the thigh, until the cylinder becomes so thick that it can be held between the thumb and finger without yielding. The surgeon now holds the cylinder in this way with the right hand, so that the portion

Fig. 42.

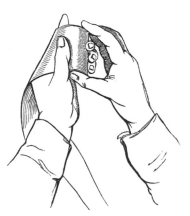

Mode of rolling a bandage by hand.

of the strip last applied is toward his face, the hand being supinated; with the thumb and forefingers of the left hand the free portion of the strip is so held as to guide it and keep it tense, as it goes to increase the cylinder, which is kept revolving by the last three fingers of the same hand, assisted by alternate pronation and supination of the right. As the muscles become fatigued in a short time by the frequent repetition of this motion, it is well to learn to perform the process with the hands reversed.

Sometimes a cylinder is made at each end of the strip of bandage, constituting what is called a double-headed roller. This is rarely used at the present day; but it may be readily formed by making one cylinder, putting in a pin to keep it from unrolling, and then making the other cylinder in the same way.

The degree of tightness with which a bandage is rolled up, whether by a machine or by the hands, will be found to influence the surgeon in his application of it; a very firm roller will be apt to be put on much more tightly than if it had been slack. Practical experience will, however, give one the faculty of judging how much pressure he is making; a bandage skilfully applied will seldom cause any annoyance by its tightness.

In putting on a bandage, the surgeon usually carries it from left to right, or from without inwards for the right arm or leg, and from within outwards for the left; especially if he be a right-handed man. He should stand in such a position as to be able to use both hands freely; facing the patient, at the extremity of the limb at first, afterwards moving, if necessary, to the side *towards* which the bandage runs. The roller, unwound to the extent of three or four inches, is held in either hand, between the thumb and the ends of the fingers, the thumb being towards the side from which the turns are to be carried, between the unwound extremity and the cylinder; the ends of the fingers, on the outside, are so near the thumb that the cylinder really lies almost in the hollow of the hand. Now, placing the outer surface of the unwound portion of the bandage

upon the skin, the surgeon fixes its initial end by putting his disengaged thumb upon it, the fingers of the
same hand passing under the limb; the hand is supine,
and the fingers embrace the limb at a lower point than
the thumb, so as not to interfere with the making of the
first turn. This first turn is generally a simple circular
one, and is sometimes repeated once so as to give additional security. Each succeeding turn should cover in
from one-third to one-half of the one before it, except
in certain special cases to be hereafter mentioned.

Fig. 43.

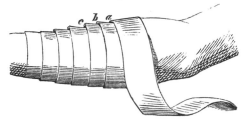

Bandage applied without reverses.

Owing to the circumstance that the limbs, as well
as the trunk, are composed of segments of cones, it is
impossible to adapt a bandage to any of them without
making what are called *reverses*. These are turns of
the bandage upon itself, so as to reverse the relation of
its surfaces to that of the limb. Supposing the surgeon
to be applying the roller to the forearm, and carrying
the turns from right to left, the outside of the roller corresponding to the surface of the skin: on reaching the
swell of the muscles, he puts his left forefinger, as in
Fig. 43, or his left thumb, as in *Fig.* 45, on the middle
of the strip, just at the point where the middle of the
reverse or fold should come; then slacking the part of

the bandage between this point and the roller, he pronates his hand so as to rotate the latter on its long axis, end for end. In this way the plane of the bandage is so changed, that it corresponds to that of the surface

Fig. 44.

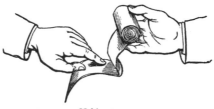

Making a reverse.

of the limb; otherwise the lower edge of each turn would stand out a little distance, while the upper edge would be closely applied. (See *Figs.* 43, 44, 45.)

Fig. 45.

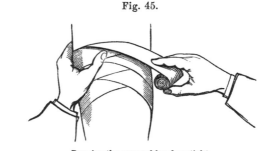

Drawing the reversed bandage tight.

When a reverse is made, it is evident that the roller will be on the inside in making the succeeding turn; and care must be taken not to let it slip from the fingers, which have a less secure hold of it in this position.

The last reverse made should bring it again to its origi-nal relation with the applied part, viz., on the outside. Every reverse should be made with a perfectly slack portion of the bandage, and drawn tight *when made;* while by keeping the edges parallel, and at equal dis-tances from one another, we may be sure of giving the whole a neat and uniform appearance. A few words must be said as to the bandaging of the upper and lower limbs respectively. In the former case, the hand and elbow-joint have to be covered in, in the latter the ankle and knee.

The initial turn of the spiral of the upper extremity is made round the wrist, the roller being then carried down across the back or palm of the hand to the fingers, the roots of which are covered by a circular turn; one or more reversed turns, according to the relative size of the hand and width of the bandage, are then made, and the wrist and thick part of the hand are covered in by figure-of-8 turns, (the mode of applying which will be presently described.) The spiral of the forearm is now put on, reverses being made to fit the swell of the mus-cles. On reaching the elbow, the surgeon again resorts to the figure-of-8, taking care to keep the joint at the precise degree of flexion to be subsequently maintained; he then resumes the circular and reversed turns until the upper arm is covered as high up as he may deem suitable.

When the lower extremity is concerned, the applica-tion of the roller is begun by one or two circular turns around the leg just above the ankle; it is then carried down across the dorsum of the foot to the root of the toes, and reversed turns made as far as the ankle, which is covered in by figure-of-8 turns crossing one another in front, when the circular and reversed turns are again employed up the leg. Arriving at the knee, the surgeon again makes figure-of-8 turns, this time crossing one another behind, in the ham, and then proceeds up the thigh with spiral reverses. Another plan is to begin by a circular turn at the root of the toes, and proceed as before.

The bandage being exhausted, or being applied to a sufficient extent, is concluded by one or two circular turns, and fastened. Some surgeons split it up for five or ten inches, and tie the two ends so formed around the limb; a method which may do very well when no pins can be had. A pin forms the best fastening; it should be neatly inserted, transversely to the strip. Other pins may be employed here and there, wherever the bandage is likely to become loosened; the heads of all these pins should be towards the upper part of the limb, so that the surgeon may pass his hand downwards over the bandage without wounding his fingers upon their points.

In taking off a bandage, the surgeon's position should be the same as in applying it. Each turn as it comes off should be gathered up with the preceding ones, so that no slack portion is left to catch anywhere and jerk the limb; and the bundle so made should be passed from one hand to the other until the whole bandage is removed.

When a bandage is much soiled, or for any reason cannot be used again, or when it is important, as in the case of large stumps, to avoid as much as possible moving the part, we may use a pair of bandage-scissors, (see *Fig.* 46,) dividing the turns of the roller instead of unwinding them.

Such is the ordinary *spiral* bandage, as used in the treatment of fractures, and whenever uniform pressure is required upon the trunk, limbs, or fingers. Any one who has learned to apply it well, can readily acquire facility in putting on any bandage whatever.

Fig. 46.

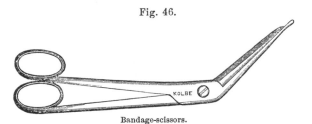

Bandage-scissors.

Where the object is merely to retain dressings, as for instance in the case of extensive burns, it will often suffice to carry the bandage much more obliquely up the limb; interspaces may be left between the several turns, and the reverses may be dispensed with. Of course much less pressure must be made in this case than in the former, lest swelling should occur in the uncovered spaces. The term *oblique* is given to bandages thus applied.

Another form in which it is often convenient to use the roller is called the *figure of-*8, or *crossed* bandage. The simplest illustration of this is the bandage employed to keep the shoulders back. Beginning at either axilla, the roller is carried up across the back to the top of the opposite shoulder, down in front of this, under the axilla, up again across the back to the top of the other shoulder, and down in front of this to the point of starting; this course being followed again and again until the desired object is sufficiently ensured, or until the roller is exhausted.   Should it be necessary to draw the shoulders forward, the same mode of application is employed,

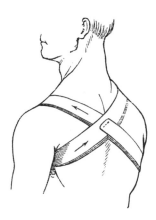

Fig. 47.

Figure-of-8 bandage of chest, (posterior.)

but the bandage is carried obliquely across the front of the chest, and down behind each shoulder. The resemblance of the figure thus described by the turns of the roller to a figure 8 needs no demonstration.

When a roller is applied in this way to a part where a limb joins the body, or to the thumb and the hand, it forms what is called a *spica* bandage; the successive turns partly covering one another, so that their junctions form a regular series of entering angles at the outer side of whatever joint may be concerned, thus producing collectively an appearance like that of the *beard* of an ear of wheat or rye.   When the lowest turn is applied first, and the roller is therefore carried upwards toward the trunk, each turn overlapping the one below it, the bandage is called an *ascending* spica.   When, on the contrary, the upper turn is first put on, and each turn overlaps that just above it, the term *descending* spica is used.

Sometimes more than two loops are made, as in Barton's bandage for fracture of the lower jaw, to be hereafter described; or as in cases where both groins are covered.

(1) A bandage of this kind is sometimes very useful

in keeping the head thrown back, as seen in *Fig.* 48. It should be 10 yards long and 2 inches wide. The head

being held in the desired position by an assistant, the surgeon begins by placing one or two circular turns from left to right around the forehead and occiput; he then carries the roller down around the back of the neck to the front of the chest, across to the left axilla, around the back to the right axilla, up over the front of the chest and around the back of the neck to the right ear; now making another circular turn, he carries the roller through the same course, and so on until the head is firmly secured.

Fig. 48.

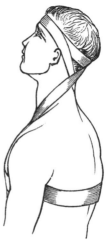

Figure-of-8 bandage of back of neck, head, and chest.

(2) When one eye is to be covered, or to have a dressing retained upon it, a figure-of-8 bandage may be applied as follows:— Use a strip 6 yards long and 1½ or 2 inches wide. If the right eye is concerned, begin at the left side,— if the left, begin at the right; carry the roller circularly once or twice around the forehead and occiput, and then, making a reverse at the latter, let the bandage go down under the ear and up over the eye of the affected side; another

Fig. 49.

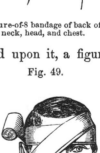

Crossed bandage of one eye.

reverse on the forehead will now make it circular, to become oblique again at the occiput. Or, which I think is a better plan, let the bandage pass up over the affected eye to a point a little above the parietal protuberance on the opposite side, and down again under the ear as before; thus encircling the head obliquely as often as may seem requisite. A few circular turns should conclude the application in either case.

(3) To cover both eyes, we may use either a single or a double-headed roller, 8 yards long and $1\frac{1}{2}$ or 2 inches wide. (a) If a single roller is used, it should be carried from left to right; one or two circular turns being made, one eye is covered as before, from below upward. Arriving at the occiput again, the roller may by a reverse be cast either upwards or downwards, so as to cover in the other eye either from above, running over the parietal protuberance of the opposite side, or from below, running under the ear of the corresponding side. Or else, having covered one eye by the method first given, the roller may by a new reverse just above the root of the nose be carried down over the other eye, under the ear, and up again to the occiput, there to become circular, and again to run the same course; a bandage so applied has however the disadvantage of being much less secure than the one previously described. Whichever is chosen, pins should be inserted wherever the bandage crosses itself, or changes its direction. (b) When a double-headed roller is employed, the central part or body is applied by its outer surface to the forehead, and the cylinders are carried round so as to meet at the occiput; with one of the cylinders we now describe one or two circular turns, and then each one is carried down from the occiput under its respective ear,

up over the corresponding eye, and to a point just above the opposite parietal protuberance, thence to the occiput again, and so on; thus forming two sets of oblique turns, crossing one another at the root of the nose and upon the occiput. The bandage last exhausted is made to describe one or two final circular turns, and the whole is secured as before by pins. Or, by making reverses, we may as in the other cases mentioned dispense with the upper parts of the oblique turns; but this plan is here also objectionable from its insecurity.

Before applying any bandage which passes over the head, especially when the patient's hair is long, it is well to put on a cap of linen or muslin; the turns of the roller are much less apt to slip if this is done. Or we may carry the last part of the bandage from before backwards in the median line, pinning it to the circular turns so as to make them sustain one another.

(4) The spica of the shoulder—crossed or figure-of-8 of the arm and chest—is sometimes used by itself, but more generally as a termination to the spiral of the arm, as will be noticed in connection with certain fractures. For this bandage we require a roller about 8 yards long, and $2\frac{1}{2}$ to 3 inches wide. Guarding the folds of the axilla by means of lint or carded cotton, we begin by making one or two circular turns from without inwards around the upper part of the arm; then carrying the bandage from the axilla up over the back and point of the shoulder, we bring it down across the front of the chest to the opposite axilla, up again across the back to the point of the shoulder, and down in front of this to the axilla where we began. By carrying the turns successively higher and higher upon the shoulder, we obtain a very neat spica.

These directions answer for the right shoulder, and also for the left if the surgeon be ambidexter, as the bandage need only in the latter case run from right to left. But it is just as well, on the left side, to carry the bandage from within outwards, up in front of the shoulder, down across the back to the opposite axilla, up across the front of the chest to the shoulder, and down behind the latter to the point of starting.

Fig. 50.

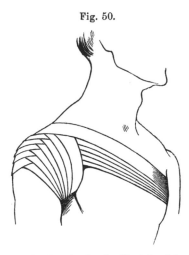

Figure-of-8 bandage of neck and axilla, (spica of shoulder.)

(5) The crossed or figure-of-8 of the neck and axilla is not very often used. A roller 5 yards long and 2 inches wide is required; one or two circular turns are made around the neck, either from before backwards or from behind forwards, and then the bandage is carried down either from the front of the neck to the back of the shoulder, or from the back of the neck to the front of the shoulder, into the axilla; hence up again,

crossing its descending portion at the side of the neck. It may be finished by a few circular turns around the upper part of the arm.

(6) The crossed or figure-of-8 of one breast is sometimes used, although it has been in a great measure superseded by adhesive strips. It consists of a roller about 10 yards long, and $2\frac{1}{2}$ inches wide. One or two circular turns having been placed around the chest, from right to left if the right breast is affected, and from left to right if the left, an oblique cast is given to the roller as it comes around to the front of the body, so as to carry it up between the breasts to the shoulder of the sound side; thence it goes down across the back, to make another circular turn, and so on, the oblique and circular turns being made alternately, and each oblique turn covering about two-thirds of the preceding one. In this way the breast may be well supported when affected with inflammation, tumors, etc.

(7) If both breasts are to be supported, a bandage at least 12 yards long, and $2\frac{1}{2}$ inches wide, will be required; it may be rolled into either one or two heads. There are several modes of procedure in these cases. (a) Several circular turns of the roller may be applied to fix it upon the chest, and then, by an oblique cast such as described in the previous paragraph, it may be carried up under one breast and down across the back. Now making another circular turn, the roller is cast obliquely upwards across the back, and down across the front of the chest under the other breast. Thus the surgeon makes four sets of turns, two circular and two oblique, the oblique crossing one another in front and behind, and so overlapping one another as to afford the necessary support and covering to both breasts. (b)

10

Another plan is to begin by carrying the roller from the right axilla up across the back to the left shoulder, down across the front of the chest, and under the right breast to the starting-point; after two or three such oblique turns, each one covering in about one-half of the preceding one, the roller is carried straight across the back to the left axilla, round under the left breast, up across the front of the chest, over the right shoulder, and down across the back to the left axilla again. One or two circular turns may serve to fix the terminal part of the bandage, and pins should be inserted at all the points of crossing. (c) A double-headed roller, of the same length and width as the single one used in the methods just detailed, may be applied for a like purpose. Placing the outer surface of the body or central portion of the bandage upon the back of the patient, carry each cylinder round to the front of her body, up under the breast, across the front of the chest to the

Fig. 51.

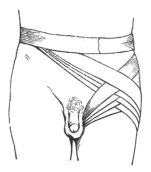

Spica or figure-of-8 bandage of groin.

shoulder; they will thus cross one another in the intermammary space; now carry each cylinder down across the back, under the axilla, up under the corresponding breast, and so on; each successive turn with each cylinder should, as in the previous methods, cover in about one-half of the foregoing one.

(8) The spica of the groin —crossed or figure-of-8 of the pelvis and thigh—requires a roller 8 or 10 yards

long and $2\frac{1}{2}$ or 3 inches wide. Make one or two circular turns around the pelvis, beginning at the crista ilii of the affected side and carrying the roller across the belly. Now, arriving again at the anterior superior spine of the ilium of the affected side, suddenly cast the roller down to the inner side of the thigh; carry it around the back of the thigh, up again across the belly, and round the back to the starting-point; make another circular turn, and then repeat the one around the inside and back of the thigh; and so on. The bandage will cross itself at the groin.

(9) If both groins are to be covered, a bandage 15 yards in length must be used. Proceed as in the other case with the circular turns, carry the roller around the root of the thigh, up again across the belly, and round the back to the point of commencement. Now carry it down across the belly, around the outer side, back, and inner side of the other thigh, up over the groin to the iliac spine, round the back, down again in front of the first groin; and so on.

(10) A spica or figure-of-8 bandage of the wrist and thumb will occasionally be found of use, either after luxations of the first metacarpal bone have been reduced, or when dressings are to be retained to the part. It requires a roller about 2 yards long and about $\frac{3}{4}$ of an inch wide. Two circular turns are first made around the wrist, beginning on its anterior surface and going from its radial to its ulnar side; the roller is then carried around the ball of the thumb, between the thumb and forefinger, back to the ulnar side of the wrist, and so on; each turn passing further and further down over the thumb.

Besides the foregoing, there are several other crossed

or figure-of-8 bandages. Some of these, as that of the chest and arm, that of the jaw, and the one known as Barton's bandage, will be described in connection with fractures. One, that of the elbow, is used in bleeding, and will be mentioned in the directions for that operation. Those of the ankle, knee, and elbow, however, are always applied in putting on the ordinary spiral bandage of the leg and arm; they need not be here detailed.

The *knotted* bandage, generally described by itself, is in reality a figure-of-8. Its

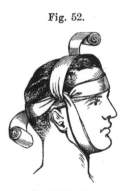

Fig. 52.

Knotted bandage.

object is to arrest hæmorrhage from the temporal artery; it is not very often used, although it might prove of great service where no other means were available. The roller employed should be a double-headed one, about 6 yards long and 1½ or 2 inches wide; one of the cylinders should be about one-third the size of the other. A compress being placed over the wound, one or two circular turns are made with the larger head of the roller around the forehead and occiput; arriving over the wound, the two portions of the bandage are knotted upon one another over the compress, and one is carried horizontally around the head, while the other goes up over its summit and down under the jaw. Meeting again over the compress, they are again knotted and again separated, and so on; the last knot terminating the application. It is obvious that this bandage, to be effectual, must be so tightly put on as to be painful; and hence it can only be temporarily used.

Recurrent bandages are employed to retain dressings upon the scalp, or to cover in stumps after amputations. When well applied, they present a very neat appearance, and are of great service. The mode of application is always the same, but a longer and wider bandage is needed for the head than for some stumps; in the former case a roller about 8 yards long and $1\frac{1}{2}$ inch wide, in the latter, if the stump is a small one, as for instance in the forearm, a roller 4 yards long and 1 inch wide. The bandage may be prepared for use either with one or two heads. (1) If a single-headed roller is used, make one or two circular turns horizontally, to fix its initial end; then on arriving at the middle of the forehead, cast the bandage directly backward over the top of the head, in the median line, to the occipital portion of the circular turns. Either pinning it here, or placing the finger of an assistant upon it, carry it forward again, a little one side of the median line, then backward, then

Fig. 53.

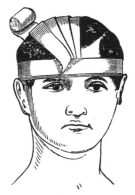

Recurrent bandage of the head.

forward, and so on, covering with each cast about one-half of the preceding one. Having come down in this way to the side of the head, carry the roller around once horizontally, and then proceed to cover in the other half of the scalp in the same manner; finishing with a few circular turns, and securing the whole by means of pins. Sometimes the terminal portion of the bandage may be carried from one side to the other over the top of the head, all the antero-posterior turns being then pinned to it. This bandage is much less secure, and hence less useful in practice, than the following. (2) If a double-headed roller is employed, the central portion of it is applied to the forehead, and both cylinders carried round to the occiput, where they cross one another, to meet again on the forehead. The lower cylinder is now carried on obliquely over the side of the head, and the upper one being carried around circularly, crosses it at the occiput and binds it down. The same thing is repeated on the other side of the head and at the forehead, and so on, the scalp being covered in symmetrically until the last two antero-posterior turns overlap one another, when a few circular turns conclude the bandage; sometimes a strip is cast across, as in the mode last detailed. The cylinder which makes the circular turns should be larger than the other by about one-half, and pins should be inserted at all the points of junction.

The recurrent bandage, as applied to stumps, varies in its length and width according to the size of the limb concerned. It may be used with either one or two heads. (1) In the former case, the initial end is carried circularly around the limb, from four to six inches above the level of the end of the bone, (the other dressings of the stump having been previously arranged;) from the posterior or lateral surface* of the limb it is

---

* From the posterior surface of the limb, when an anterior and a posterior flap are made, or when after a circular operation the lips of the wound are brought together transversely; from the lateral surface when the wound is closed in a vertical line after the circular amputation, or when two lateral flaps are made. In other words, the recurrent turns should cross the wound at right angles.

reflected down over the end of the stump, up to the anterior part of the circular turns, back again, and so

Fig. 54.

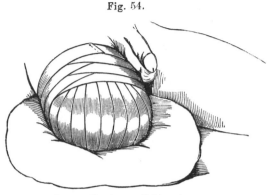

Recurrent bandage applied to a stump.

on, just as has been already directed in regard to the head. The terminal portion of the bandage may be carried up the limb as a spiral. Sometimes, especially if the stump be one of large size, the roller is reversed so as to form a circular turn after each recurrent, each circular overlapping the preceding one by about two-thirds; in this way we avoid the inconvenience of an accumulation of circular turns at one portion of the limb. (2) The double-headed roller is not often used for the recurrent bandage of a stump, the single-headed being equally efficient and more readily applied; when the former is employed, however, the method of putting it on is exactly the same as for the head, and need not be here repeated.

Invaginated bandages are such as are made to terminate in two or more tails, which are to be passed through corresponding openings, either in the same or in another strip; the object being that the perforated and the perforating portions may act in exactly opposite directions, holding the lips of the wound together through the medium of compresses. The tails, thus carried through the corresponding openings, may be best secured by pinning them separately; although some writers direct that they should be kept in place simply by the succeeding turns of the roller. M. Gerdy[*] has proposed what he calls the invaginated spiral bandage, for longitudinal wounds of the trunk or limbs. The following rules for applying it to a limb will sufficiently exhibit the principle involved. A double-headed roller about two inches wide, and as long as may be deemed necessary, with compresses and any other suitable dressings, are provided; the limb is enveloped in a spiral from the fingers or toes upward as far as the wound; now, placing the body of the double-headed roller upon the opposite side of the limb from the wound, and arranging the compresses, etc. in place, the surgeon directs an assistant to make a longitudinal slit close to one head of the roller, large enough to admit of the other head passing through it. Crossing the ends in this way, he now carries them round to a little above the starting-point, and crossing them here by a simple reverse, brings them back over the wound, where the slitting process is again resorted to, and so on; the two ends being finally pinned or tied together.

Perhaps the *many-tailed* bandages may be as appropriately described here as at any other time. They may consist of a number of strips independent of one

---

[*] Traité des Bandages, p. 176. Paris, 1837.

another, or of a single piece of muslin slit up at its margins or extremities. The latter form will for the sake of convenience be first described.

(1) The many-tailed bandage of the head, called also the *poor man's bandage*, or *bandage of Galen*, is designed to retain dressings upon the scalp. It consists of a central portion or body, and of three tails on each side. The central portion being applied, the two posterior tails are brought forward and tied together upon the forehead; the two anterior ones are carried backward to meet over the occiput, while the two middle ones go downward to meet under the chin.

(2) The many-tailed bandage of the chin is smaller than the foregoing, and its mode of application is exactly the converse. Its body being placed upon the chin, its posterior tails meet over the front part of the top of the head, its anterior tails go backward to meet over the occiput, its middle ones come together at the vertex. This bandage may also be made with only two tails on a side, as in the annexed cut. (See *Fig*. 55.)

Fig. 55.

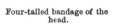

Four-tailed bandage of the head.

(3) The many-tailed bandage of the shoulder has either two or three tails on each side. Its body being placed over the shoulder, its upper tails, shorter than the others, go directly downwards to meet under the axilla; the next pair pass one in front and the other behind the chest, to meet in the opposite axilla, and the lowest pair, which are often dispensed with, pass up to meet on the opposite side of the neck.

Other applications of this species of bandage may be very easily devised upon occasion, for the elbow, knee, heel, etc.

(4) The bandage of Scultetus comes properly under this head, and will therefore be here described. It consists of a number of strips long enough to go once and a half around the part affected, and of any desired width; these may either be arranged on a pillow or a board to be slipped under the limb, or laid in order upon the bed, and the limb then let down upon them. The strip which is to come nearest the trunk should be first laid down, the next should overlap it about one-third, and so on; when they are applied to the limb, this order will of course be reversed, the strip furthest from the trunk being the one first put on, and the limb being covered in from below upward. Either the upper or lower extremity may be thus enveloped in its entire length. When one or more of the strips become soiled, the bandage may be turned aside as far as may be necessary, and then, pinning a clean strip to the end of each soiled one, we may draw the latter out, and by the same movement bring its substitute in. In this way the limb will be much less disturbed than it would have to be in applying a fresh roller.—Another plan is to use a single piece of muslin, of any desired length, and wide enough to go once and a half around the limb; the lateral margins being slit up to within an inch or two of the median line, so that the strips are connected by a central portion from two to four inches in width. Convenient as this method would be in many respects, it has not the advantage of allowing us to change soiled portions of the dressing in the manner before detailed.

Bandages in the shape of the letter T are often useful, for the purpose of retaining dressings to various parts. They of course vary much in size, for the different portions of the body; it may also be convenient to use two or more vertical pieces instead of only one. The several parts are generally sewed together, but they may be attached to one another quite as well by means of pins.

A few only of the applications of this form of bandage need be mentioned here; a little ingenuity on the part of the surgeon will enable him to adapt it in special cases.

(1) To retain dressings upon the scalp, the T bandage may often be substituted with advantage for the more complex recurrent. For this purpose we require a transverse band from one to two yards long and one inch wide, to which we attach a vertical portion of equal width, but only half as long, or somewhat less. The central part of the transverse band being placed on the forehead, just above the root of the nose, the vertical strip is carried up over the top of the head in the median line, so as to hang down at the back of the neck; now the ends of the transverse band are brought around and crossed over the occiput, confining the vertical one at this point; the latter is now folded back upon itself, and meets the two ends of the former again upon the forehead, where a pin may be used to secure them all; if the extremities are too long, they may be cut off close. Sometimes it may be well to add another strip across the top of the head, pinning it to the transverse band above the ear on each side, and to the vertical one at the top of the head.

(2) To retain dressings upon the nose, the transverse

band, about half an inch wide, should pass over the
upper lip and round to the back of the head; two other
bands of the same width, sewed to the former so as to
form with it a triangle just large enough to take in the
nose, run up from it, crossing at the root of the organ,
and meeting again at the occiput, where they are confined by the transverse band, looped around it, and
knotted together; the ends of the transverse band cross
one another, and one of them is carried around above
the ear, across the forehead, to meet its fellow above
the other ear, when they are knotted together.

(3) When dressings are to be retained upon or behind
the ear, a T bandage may be of great service. The
transverse piece, about a yard and a half long, and
three-quarters of an inch wide, should have a piece of
about the size and shape of the dressing sewed to its
lower edge; this piece terminating below in the vertical
strip, which should be of the same width as the transverse, and somewhat longer. The central piece being
duly arranged, the vertical strip is carried down under
the jaw, up over the opposite temple, and down again
to be pinned to the transverse band; the ends of the
latter are passed around the head, cross one another
above the opposite ear, confining the vertical strip, and
come back again to be tied over the point of commencement.

(4) Bandages applied around the thorax are very apt
to slip downwards; those around the abdomen and pelvis are very apt to slip upwards. Hence pieces are
added to pass up over the shoulders or down under the
perineum, constituting true T bandages; the principle
involved is too simple to call for any further detail.

(5) Sometimes it is necessary to keep dressings ap-

plied to the palm or back of the hand; and for this
purpose we might employ a band around the wrist,
with other bands passing from it between the fingers.
But for obvious reasons it is better to attach to the
transverse band a piece, as wide as the hand, and somewhat more than twice as long as the distance from the
lower edge of the band to the roots of the fingers;

Fig. 56.

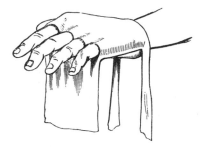

doubling this over, we cut out at the fold holes fitted to
receive the fingers; now applying the dressing, we pass
the fingers through the holes, bring the free end of the
vertical piece up to the wrist, make the circular turn
around the wrist, and pin the whole securely. Such a
bandage is called the perforated T of the hand. A
modification of this bandage might be employed for the
foot; but generally speaking, either for the foot or the
hand, an ordinary roller will be found quite as effectual,
and much more easy of application.

Handkerchief bandages, in their simpler forms, are
very commonly used in domestic surgery; they have
been brought into notice as scientific appliances chiefly

11

by M. Mathias Mayor, of Lausanne, in Switzerland, who has very carefully systematized them.*

The main principle involved in M. Mayor's system of bandaging, is the derivation of various confining means from a square piece of muslin or linen, as large as a pocket-handkerchief, or larger if need be. M. Gerdy† places the different forms of bandage thus obtained under the head of "*entire* bandages," (*plein,*) because they do not involve division of the stuff composing them; but the term proposed by M. Mayor, which has been adopted in this chapter, is clearer and more suggestive. The advantages of this system, as well as the objections to it, will be mentioned in connection with its special applications; suffice it to say at present, that it has not yet fulfilled the anticipations of its ingenious author, by superseding all other methods of bandaging. I shall now endeavor to give the reader an idea of its main features.

For surgical purposes, a handkerchief may be used as such, or it may be folded in either one of four ways. (1) It may be so doubled upon itself as to constitute a long quadrangular band. (2) Its opposite angles may be brought together, so as to form the apex of a triangle, the base of which corresponds to the diagonal of the primitive square. To this apex the name of *summit* or *point* is given, the other angles being called *extremities*, and the side opposite the summit retaining the name of *base*. (3) The triangle may be folded on itself so as to resemble the ordinary cravat, with two

---

* Bandages et Appareils à Pansements, ou Nouveau Systéme de Déligation Chirurgicale. Paris, 1832.

† Op. cit. p. 152.

extremities and a central portion or *body*. (4) A cord may be formed by twisting the cravat upon itself.

I. THE HANDKERCHIEF.—This is used for only one purpose, viz., to cover in the head. Fold it so that one margin shall approach within about two inches of the opposite one; let the fold come at the back of the neck, the longer portion being next the head; tie the two anterior corners of the outer portion under the chin, and then draw out the corners of the inner portion as much as possible from beneath the outer; turn back the excess of the inner portion over the outer, and knot the corners of the former below the occiput.

II. THE OBLONG.—This is used for making a sling for the forearm, which is placed upon the middle of it, the two ends being brought up and pinned together to the front of the coat or dress. It may also, when long enough, be used to make a circular of the thorax or abdomen; or it may be employed to retain dressings to any of the limbs.

III. TRIANGLES.—These may be divided into the *caps*, intended to cover in the whole of a rounded part, such as the head, the buttock, or a stump, and the *triangles*, intended simply to give support, and only covering the part in order to ensure firmness.

(1) The cap for covering the scalp is very simple. (*a*) The base of a triangle being placed over the forehead, its summit hanging down at the back of the neck, the two extremities are carried round, crossed posteriorly so as to confine the summit, brought back again to the forehead, and there tied or pinned; the summit is

now turned up to be fastened to the portion covering the scalp. (*b*) The relations of the triangle to the occiput and forehead may be reversed. But the knot must not be placed at the occiput, as its pressure would be injurious; the ends should be crossed there, and secured further round by means of pins.

(2) The cap of the breast is thus made:—Place the base of the triangle just below the affected organ, carrying one extremity under the adjoining axilla, and the other over the opposite shoulder, so that they meet upon the back; the summit, passing up over the clavicle of the affected side, is now to be passed beneath the dorsal portion and secured. When the diseased breast is of large size, this bandage may be of great use in supporting it, as well as in retaining dressings upon it.

(3) (*a*) Both buttocks may readily be covered by placing the base of the triangle over the lumbar vertebræ, carrying the extremities round to meet over the abdomen, and passing the summit forwards between the thighs, so that it may be brought up and fastened in the usual way. (*b*) When only one buttock is concerned, the base of the triangle is placed over the great trochanter, the extremities carried around the thigh, and the summit attached to a cravat or other girdle around the loins.

(4) The testicles may be covered and supported as follows:—A cravat is first tied about the loins. The base of a small triangle being now placed behind the scrotum, its two extremities are carried up in front of the cravat, passed beneath it, brought out on each side a little distance from the median line, and tied together; the summit is now carried up under this knot, under the cravat, turned down again, and fastened by tying or

pinning. This bandage answers the same purpose as the suspensory of the testicles, to be hereafter described; it may be stitched up if necessary so as to fit the part more accurately.

Fig. 57.

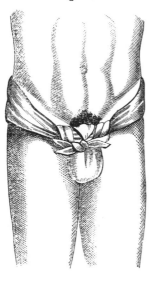

Fig. 58.

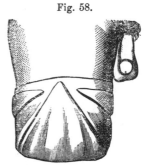

(5) Stumps may be covered by a triangle arranged exactly as for the head, the knot being of course made to come upwards. The objection to this bandage is the readiness with which it becomes deranged.

Analogous applications of the triangle to the hand, heel, foot, etc., may be readily contrived. The other mode of employing it is much less important in practice, if we except the sling, which in its various forms is constantly found useful; it may, however, be very valuable to the surgeon, where circumstances render his ordinary resources unavailable, and hence cannot be altogether neglected here.

(a) The *oculo-occipital* triangle, intended to cover both eyes, is applied by very much the same rules as the cap

11*

for the scalp, the only difference being that in the present case the body of the triangle is placed lower down, and always of course anteriorly.

(*b*) The *occipito-sternal* triangle is intended to draw the head forward. A cravat being tied around the chest, with its body in front, the body of a triangle is applied to the top of the head, and its extremities brought down, one on each side of the face, to be fastened to the cravat over the sternum. Such an arrangement might serve a temporary purpose, but could not be relied upon as a permanency. The *fronto-dorsal* triangle is exactly the reverse of the preceding, in its object and mode of application. The *parieto-axillary* is intended to draw the head down sideways, its body being placed upon the parietal region, and its extremities knotted in the opposite axilla.

(*c*) The *thoracico-scapulary* triangle is used to retain dressings at the upper and lateral portions of the back. The body of the triangle being placed just below the part to be covered, its two extremities are brought round the chest and tied together at the opposite point; the summit is then brought over either shoulder as the case may be, to be directly or indirectly attached to the portion in front of the chest.

(*d*) The *cruro-inguinal* triangle is meant to supply the place of the figure-of-8 bandage of the groin, but is much less secure. Placing the base of the bandage obliquely behind the pelvis, from above downwards toward the affected side, the surgeon carries the lower extremity round in front of the groin, to the inner side of the thigh, behind it, round again on its outer side, and back to the fold of the groin. The summit is brought forward between the thighs, and up to be attached to the first extremity in front of the groin; while the upper extremity of the triangle runs up behind the pelvis, round it, and down to be attached over the groin of the affected side.

(e) A *sling for the arm* may be made with a triangle

Fig. 59.

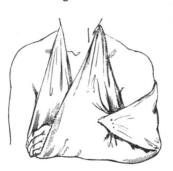

Sling for the arm, made with one handkerchief folded triangularly.

in several ways. The best mode is to tie a cravat loosely around the neck, with the knot in front; then, placing the base of the triangle under the wrist, pass one of its extremities through the cravat, and tie the other to it; finally, bring the summit well up back of the elbow, cast it forward, and pin it so as to support the elbow effectively.—The cravat may very often be dispensed with, the two extremities of the triangle passing up on each side of the neck to be knotted together behind it; but it is evidently useful in preventing the pressure of the knot upon the skin.—The base of the triangle being placed below the hand, one extremity may be carried round under the corresponding axilla to the back, and thence up to the opposite shoulder, there to meet the other extremity brought directly up in front; the summit may be brought round in front of the arm to be secured as in the other method.—Another excellent plan is as follows:—Pass the base of the triangle up under the arm to be supported; tie its extremities at the opposite side or upon the back, bring the summit up over the opposite shoulder and down the back to be secured to the other portion, either immediately or by means of a strip. If the elbow needs especial support, the slack edge of the handkerchief around it may be taken up and fastened with a pin.

IV. CRAVATS.—These are less useful than the foregoing, being very apt indeed to become deranged, unless applied with a degree of tightness which in some parts of the body would cause injurious pressure. Either one or several may be required in any special case, as a temporary expedient.

(1) The *fronto-occipito-labial* cravat is applied by placing its body upon the forehead, crossing its extremities over the occiput, again crossing them, or passing one through a slit out in the other, over the upper lip, and tying or pinning the ends near the ears.

(2) The *bis-axillary* cravat is intended to retain dressings in the axilla, by the pressure of its body; its two extremities being carried up, one in front and the other behind, to cross one another at the top of the shoulder, and thence to go down across the chest and back, to meet and be knotted in the opposite axilla. Here, as elsewhere, care should be taken to guard the points likely to suffer from pressure.

(3) The *cruro-inguinal* cravat, applied exactly like the triangle of the same name, except that it has of

course no summit to be passed forwards between the thighs, answers the same purpose.

(4) The *sacro-bicrural* cravat is applied by placing its body just above the sacrum, carrying each extremity round in front of the corresponding groin, down upon the perineum, and up again round the back and outside of the thigh of the same side, to be secured at the groin.

Many other applications of the cravat may be found useful in special cases. M. Mayor, and others following him, have proposed the employment of it for suspending the foot, for confining the hand to the upper arm, etc. As temporary expedients, such arrangements may answer very well, but they have the inconvenience of causing congestion and swelling of the parts below, since they constrict the limb circularly, and of course hinder the passage of venous blood. Cravats are among the most important constituents of M. Mayor's apparatus for almost every fracture; but they must, in order to act efficiently in such cases, be applied quite firmly, and hence involve more or less risk of the unpleasant consequence above referred to.

V. THE CORD.—This form of the handkerchief bandage is very seldom used, being apt by the unevenness of its surface to injure the skin. When hæmorrhage occurs from a wound of the femoral or brachial artery, a cord may be used in making what is called the Spanish windlass, which has been described with the other means for the arrest of bleeding; but a cravat answers the same purpose.

Such are the main features of M. Mayor's system, so far as regards the substitution of handkerchiefs for ordinary bandages; the peculiarities of his method of treating fractures and other injuries will be more appropriately mentioned elsewhere.

Another system of bandaging has been proposed by M. Rigal de Gaillac, at the *Académie de Médecine* in Paris. His plan is to use triangles, etc., connected with one another by means of caoutchouc bands; the idea being that the elasticity of the latter will obviate the liability of the apparatus to derangement by the movements of the part. It is hardly worth while to enter into detail here with regard to this system, which is not likely to come into general use; in any case where its peculiarities would render it specially available, a little contrivance would enable the surgeon to carry out the idea.

SHEATHS are used to protect the penis, fingers or toes from the friction of the clothes, or from the air; if necessary, a poultice might be applied in this way. When, however, it is desirable to retain dressings upon the parts alluded to, the difficulty is to put the sheath on without disturbing the former. It is, therefore, better to answer the purpose by taking a piece of soft linen or muslin, four or five times as wide as the diameter of the part to be protected, and exceeding it in length by from one-third to one-half. Having arranged the other dressings upon the part, apply one margin of the piece which is to form the sheath as high up as may be requisite; fold over the surplus length of the piece, and then envelop the part in its lateral portions; a narrow bandage, or a few stitches, may serve to secure the sheath thus made.

SUSPENSORIES are mainly used in cases of varicocele, cirsocele, epididymitis, orchitis, or other diseases of the male genitals. Their office is sufficiently indicated by their name.

An apparatus of this kind may be readily obtained of almost any instrument-maker or apothecary. But it is evidently much better that the surgeon should construct a suspensory of exactly the proper size and shape, or at least that he should be able to do so in case of need. For this purpose, a piece of soft muslin or linen, of oblong shape and any required size, should be applied by one of its longer margins behind the scrotum, so that the adjacent margins may be brought together in front of it, overlapping a little. The double edge thus formed is cut away in a curved line, towards its upper end, so as to form a rounded opening to accommodate the penis, the lower corner so that a central seam shall run up the under and anterior surface of the scrotum; the posterior surface being fitted by a similar cutting away of the lower part of the fold. The seam should be made on the outside, so as not to cut the skin. Tapes are attached to each side of the front part of the bag so formed, and to its posterior part so as to run beneath the perineum, both sets coming up to a band around the waist, to be secured by buttoning, tying or pinning.

Besides this suspensory there are two others, one for the breast and the other for the nose. The latter is very easily made by cutting out a piece of muslin or linen so as to fit the nose, attaching one band to its upper extremity to run up over the head in the median line, and other bands to its lateral corners to pass circularly around the head, just below the ears, to be tied together and confine the posterior extremity of the first-named band at the occiput.

For retaining dressings to the breast, or for supporting that organ when it is very large, as in cases of abscess or other disease, a suspensory may be employed. A square piece of linen or muslin, large enough to cover the affected part, is laid upon the latter, and its surplus gathered in folds from each corner toward the centre. Cutting these folds away, we have what is well known as the Maltese cross; now by sewing the cut edges together, we form a somewhat closely-fitting cap, which may be kept in place over the breast by four tapes, two fastened to the upper corners of the cap and tied behind the neck, two to the lower corners and tied behind the chest.

CHAPTER VII.

FRACTURES.

THESE injuries are invariably the result of mechanical violence; hence they most frequently affect the long bones, and the most exposed of these, as the humerus, clavicle, femur, and bones of the leg. A force and a resistance are necessary, according to the laws of mechanics; blows, falls, crushing, and inordinate muscular contraction are the chief causes by which bones are broken.

When the force acts at the point of lesion, the resistance being at both ends of the bone, the fracture is said to be by direct violence. But when the force is applied at one end and the resistance at the other, the bone giving way at some intermediate point, the fracture is said to be by indirect violence.

Some persons are predisposed to fracture, by the inherent fragility of their osseous system; the old are so, by the natural changes in form as well as in composition of their bones. Some follow occupations which expose them to violence; and some are affected with cancer or other local disease of the bone which gives way.

Pain, loss of power, swelling and ecchymosis, are apt to attend fracture of any bone; but the reliable symp-

12 (129)

toms are deformity and preternatural mobility at the
seat of injury, and above all, crepitation when the
broken ends are moved one upon another.

All fractures are

SIMPLE or COMPOUND;
either of which may be
Complete or Incomplete;

(In long bones,)		(In flat bones,)
Transverse,	(In either)	Fissured,
Oblique, or	comminuted,	Stellate, or
Longitudinal.	complicated, or both.	Camerated.

(In the bones of the skull) depressed.

Simple fractures are such as do not communicate
with the atmosphere by a wound. *Compound* fractures
are such as do so communicate. Abscess or gangrene
may convert a simple into a compound fracture.

Complete fractures are such as involve the entire
thickness of the bone affected. The terms *transverse,
oblique, longitudinal, fissured,* and *stellate,* explain
themselves. *Camerated* fractures always affect flat or
thick bones; they present several cracks radiating from
a depressed point. *Comminuted* fractures are those in
which there are more than two fragments.

Complicated fractures are such as have associated
with them other serious lesions, such as dislocation, injury of nerves, blood-vessels or viscera. The term is
usually applied only when the superadded hurt is in
the neighborhood of the affected bone.

After a simple fracture is sustained, inflammation is
set up at the seat of injury, and subsides only after the
lapse of six or eight days, or in some cases later. It
gradually gives place to the reparative process; and

this, being completed roughly in from three to eight weeks, the *modelling* of the new material by absorption begins, and lasts for an indefinite time. Some cases give scarcely any trouble after the first dressing, recovery taking place with hardly any impairment of function or perceptible deformity. Occasionally, however, we meet with cases of *delayed union*, and more rarely with those of *non-union* or *false-joint.*

A simple fracture, painful as it may be, is not apt to involve any danger, except in very old or feeble persons. Compound fracture, especially in the lower extremities, is more serious; the shock to the system is greater, and the patient has to run the subsequent risk of inflammation, suppuration, tetanus, and hectic fever. Complicated fractures, of course, are more or less grave according to the character of the complication. A fracture near a joint is very apt to be followed by a greater or less degree of stiffening, even though the joint be not involved in the first injury. Of this the surgeon should always be careful to forewarn the patient and his friends, lest fault be found with the treatment when an unsatisfactory result ensues. Much trouble may be saved in this way. Moreover, every fracture is apt to leave behind it some degree of stiffness of the limb, with a tendency to rheumatic pains, aggravated by atmospheric changes; and these unavoidable sequelæ of the injury may be charged to defects in the treatment, unless the surgeon has predicted them from the outset.

When called to any case of fracture, the surgeon has to consider certain questions. As in every other instance, the general condition of the patient must first be looked to; a few cheerful words may allay his mental agitation, and alcoholic stimulus or a sedative may be needed to steady his shaken nerves.* If away from home, the question of removal must be considered; and if the measure be decided upon, arrangements must be made for effecting it with the least possible delay or inconvenience. In grave cases, and especially when the lower extremity is injured, this is a matter of serious moment. In military practice, the question of amputation sometimes turns upon the distance the sufferer must be carried, and the available means for transporting him.

Carrying by hand is always best, unless prevented by the distance to be gone over, or the want of men. The bearers selected should be as nearly as possible of the same height, and should *not* keep step with one another. They should stop at proper intervals, to let the patient rest as well as themselves; in very bad cases it is well also for the surgeon to examine occasionally as to the need of renewed stimulus, or of any other attention. In military and hospital practice, a *stretcher*, or litter of canvas stretched upon poles, is generally used; in civil life, a settee or shutter, covered with bed-quilts or blankets. On an emergency, an army surgeon may direct two soldiers to fasten a blanket between two muskets for the purpose.

Armies are also supplied with *ambulances* for one, two or four horses; and litters arranged to be placed upon the back of a horse or mule have been employed.

---

* The surgeon must use his judgment about these matters; f℥ss of brandy, whiskey, or any available liquor, with or without water, may be given at once or in divided doses; or the ammoniated tincture of valerian, Hoffman's anodyne, spirits of camphor, opium in any of its preparations, when a more exclusively calming influence seems to be called for.

The latter are more available for convalescents or slightly injured men than for grave cases. Four-wheeled wagons are found to be decidedly better than two-wheeled, as regards the comfort of the wounded. Mule-litters, or *cacolets*, were found more useful than either in the Crimean war.* With the details of these contrivances we are not now concerned; but under all circumstances the surgeon's first duty is to arrange the injured limb so as to protect it as far as possible from any derangement of the broken ends of the bone. If he can, he should lay the patient on a hard and even mattress, or on a flat bed of folded quilts, or of straw; but at any rate the limb should be well and firmly supported.

The surgeon had better himself take charge of the lifting of the broken limb, as in private practice he generally can. On arriving at the house, he should examine the passages and stairways, and the arrangement of the room and bed, so as to determine how best to have the patient brought in; for want of this foresight, much inconvenience may ensue. When the fracture is a severe one of the arm or forearm, and the patient suffers much from shock, it is best for the surgeon to carry the injured member, while the rest of the body and the lower limbs are sustained by a sufficient number of attendants. In slighter cases, the arm may be merely suspended in a sling; while sometimes the patient is able to walk perfectly well, with the injured member either laid in a sling or carried in the opposite hand.

The best plan, when it is the lower extremity that is involved, is for an assistant on either side to support

---

* Delafield's Report on the Art of War in Europe, p. 73. (1861.)

the pelvis with one hand and the shoulders with the other, the patient putting an arm around each of their necks ; another assistant may lift the sound limb, while the surgeon carries the injured one. A child or a very light adult may be carried by one assistant. A very heavy person may need three or four ; it is always better to have too much force employed than too little.

On coming into the room, if the settee is brought in, it should be set down with its open side towards the bed, in such a way that the patient may be transferred directly to the latter ; one or two strong assistants standing over him to lift him, and the surgeon still having charge of the broken limb. If the patient be carried in the arms, the assistants should either go one on each side of the bed, and so lay him down upon it ; or he may be seated on the edge of the bed, and then, one assistant getting on the bed and the others lifting at the side, he may be turned and laid down. As a general rule, at first at least, the injured limb should be nearest the edge of the bed, if the latter be a wide one.

Proper measures should of course be taken beforehand to prevent any soiling of the bedclothes or sheets, whether by the feet of assistants, by dirt on the clothes of the patient, or by blood from the wound if there be one.

Much pain may be saved the patient by ripping or cutting his clothes off, instead of removing them in the usual way, for the examination of the injury ; the boots particularly, in a fracture of the leg or thigh, should be slit up, and not pulled off. The use of anæsthetics will not only save the patient pain during the examination, but will very often enable the surgeon to arrive at a far more satisfactory knowledge of the nature of the case he has to deal with; they should be resorted to without hesitation unless contraindicated by the existence of visceral disease.

In every case of fracture, reduction should be permanently effected at the earliest possible moment; if the patient has to be transported a long distance, it is all the more important for his comfort and safety that the limb should be properly secured for the journey. This reduction, or "setting," is popularly thought to involve extreme pain; but in fact, if well performed, it rather gives relief than otherwise. It is effected by gentle but firm traction on either end of the bone, with coaptation or fitting of the fragments; the surgeon may or may not need assistance, according to the size of the bone involved.

In the treatment of fractures, the surgeon has to bear in mind carefully the forms and relations of the bones concerned, and any peculiarities they may present in different patients should be noticed. Thus the humerus and femur, as well as the ulna and tibia, are in one aspect directly subcutaneous; and if pressure can be made first along these surfaces, it will be more effective than if exerted through an intervening mass of muscular tissue. Again, some men have a much greater degree of curvature than others in the outlines of all their long bones; and this must be allowed for.

Before any apparatus is put on, it will often be clearly indicated, and will always be comfortable to the patient, that the injured limb should be thoroughly cleansed with soap and warm water. This operation ought to be done by the surgeon himself, unless he has a skilful assistant, upon whose care and gentleness he can depend. A fine soft sponge is the best means of applying the water, and much pain will be saved by the use of a soft old towel in the drying of the part. This washing should be repeated at intervals of one or two days during the whole course of the treatment, the cure being actually favored by a wholesome state of the skin. The details of the process will be given in connection with each fracture. Anæsthetics are often required in the operation, and should be employed in all suitable cases.

SPECIAL FRACTURES.

§ 1.—FRACTURES OF THE SKULL.

These injuries are chiefly important from the danger they involve to the brain and its membranes. Any special symptoms arising from them demand either energetic medical treatment, or perhaps the operation of trephining; neither of which come within the scope of the present work.

§ 2.—FRACTURES OF THE BONES OF THE FACE.

Fractures of the Nasal Bones are always caused by direct violence, such as a blow or kick. The deformity and pain are very great; sometimes, especially if the cribriform plate of the ethmoid bone has been broken, inflammation of the brain may arise, and destroy life.

The treatment is to pass a female catheter, a quill, or some instrument of like shape, up the nostril, and mould the bones upon it; lint wet with ice-water being afterwards kept constantly applied until the pain and inflammation have subsided. Depletory medical treatment is also called for in most cases.

When the nasal cartilages are broken or displaced, the symptoms and treatment are the same as in the former case.

Fractures of the Upper Maxillary Bone are always caused by great and direct violence, such as gunshot, or the kick of a horse; they are very apt to be compound. In most cases of this kind the chief danger is from hæmorrhage; the vessel should be sought for and ligatured, if possible; if it cannot be found, strong styptics should be made use of; and if these fail, the wound must be well cleansed by sponging or syringing, and the actual cautery applied. Cold water-dressings will generally afford most comfort.

When the alveolar process is involved, and especially if the fracture is confined to it, the teeth on either side of the injury ought to be fastened together by means of a wire loop cast around them. It is usually better for the wire to embrace four teeth; its ends are drawn as tightly as seems proper, twisted together, cut off, and a little bit of cork or gutta-percha stuck on so as to prevent them from scratching the mucous membrane of the cheek.

Deformity can scarcely be avoided after these injuries.

Fractures of the Lower Jaw are caused by direct violence. The part of the bone most frequently affected is the body, but it may give way at any point. Sometimes, especially in compound fractures from gunshot, there may be a number of fragments. The signs of the injury are seldom obscure, the fragments being generally much displaced by the contraction of the numerous muscles inserted into them. By passing one or two fingers into the mouth, the others being applied outside the chin, we can in most cases ascertain the exact character of the lesion.

Fig. 60.

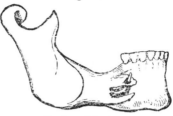

Fracture of the jaw.

Much care is required in the treatment of this injury. The beard, if the patient wears one, should first be

Fig. 61.

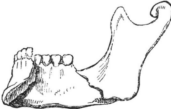

Double fracture of the jaw.

shaved entirely off. If there is great displacement, or if, although slight, it tends to recur, the teeth should be wired together as in the case of the upper jaw; then, care being taken to make the lower dental arch correspond to the upper, a pasteboard or gutta-percha cap (*Fig.* 62) should be fitted to the chin. Sometimes a very small firm compress, so placed as to bear against the inner border of the lower jaw, is of use in preventing either fragment from projecting inwards. The cap being held in place by adhesive strips passing round beneath and in front of it, is then firmly bound on by means of the following bandage, first described by Dr. Barton. A roller 2 inches wide and 7 yards long is applied, commencing below the occiput, passing up over the parietal protuberance, across the sagittal suture, down the side of the face, under the chin, up the other side of the face, and across the top of the head again to below the occiput;

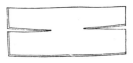

Fig. 62.

Pasteboard or gutta-percha cap for fracture of the lower jaw.

two ovals being thus made, a third is added by a turn along under the ear, in front of the chin, and back again under the other ear. This process being repeated until the roller is exhausted, pins are placed at all the points of intersection. Nothing can be more elegant or effective than this bandage when neatly and firmly put on. (See *Fig.* 63.)

Another plan is to slit up a bandage, 3 inches wide and

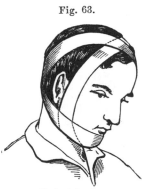

Fig. 63.

Barton's bandage.

a yard in length, from either end to within 3 inches of the centre; which being applied over the jaw, the two tails on either side are crossed over one another, and the corresponding ones tied at the top and back of the head respectively. (See *Fig.* 55.)

Various machines, with plates to fit the dental arch and the under part of the jaw, have been devised; they hardly admit of any general description, within our present limits.* Very often, however, the surgeon may accomplish the same end by taking a piece of gutta-percha or sheet-lead, doubling it over upon itself, bending it to make it fit the dental arch, and leaving it thus in position when the outside cap and the bandage are put on. If necessary, both the upper and lower dental arches may be thus confined.

¿ 3.—FRACTURES OF THE BONES OF THE TRUNK.

Fractures of the Vertebræ are generally the result of falls, or of some crushing force, such as the passage of a wagon wheel over the body. In the former case, the injury may actually be due to indirect violence, the bone giving way before the momentum of one portion of the body, the other being suddenly checked by contact with the ground, or with some other obstacle. The symptoms vary much according to the point at which the vertebral column gives way; and depend for their importance upon the injury inflicted on the spinal marrow and the nerves given off from at and below the spot. The cord may be broken through, lacerated, or

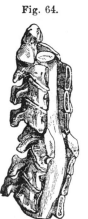

Fig. 64.

Fracture of cervical vertebræ with displacement.

---

* For descriptions of such contrivances, the reader is referred to the voluminous treatises of Malgaigne and Hamilton.

pressed upon; the pressure being caused either by displacement of the fragments, or by effusion of blood, serum, or lymph beneath the membranes. Sometimes the patient seems to do very well until, by some inadvertent motion, the fragments are thrown out of place.

Loss of sensation and voluntary motion, irregular pains, and abnormities of temperature, with paralysis of the muscular coats of the bowel or bladder, or of the sphincters, are the main symptoms.

The treatment of these cases consists chiefly in promoting comfort, and in endeavoring to correct and obviate whatever troubles may arise. Great care should be taken in the lifting and handling of the patient, and in the examination of the injury. Pillows and compresses should be so arranged on a firm mattress as to support the whole body in the easiest posture. If involuntary discharges take place from the bladder and rectum, the bed should be duly protected. Bed-sores are very apt to occur, and must be guarded against by stimulation of the skin, by air-cushions, changes of position, etc. Particular attention must be paid to drawing off the urine as it collects, by means of the catheter; the bowels must also be unloaded from time to time, by cathartics or enemata.

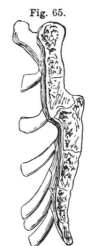

Fig. 65.

Fracture of the sternum.

Fractures of the Sternum are generally due to severe blows, to the kick of a horse, or to crushing force; but cases are on record in which the bone has been forced asunder by great muscular effort

13

on the part of the patient. They are attended with
great pain, and usually with deformity; mediastinal abscess and caries of the bone have sometimes ensued.
Immediate death has been caused in some of the cases
by injury of the heart.

Careful adjustment of the fragments, a firm bandage
around the chest, with anodyne and antiphlogistic measures, must be resorted to; and any complications must
be carefully watched for and promptly met.

Fig. 66.

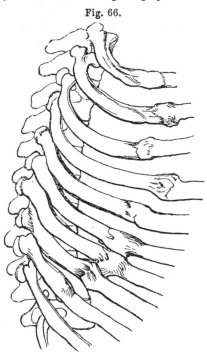

Fracture involving eight ribs.

Fractures of the Ribs may be caused by direct violence, or by the application of crushing force tending to

increase the curvature of the bones. Great pain and difficulty in breathing, with deformity and crepitus, are the principal symptoms. Emphysema, pneumothorax, pleurisy, and pneumonia may any or all of them ensue.

A firm bandage round the chest, or the application of a sufficient number of adhesive strips to support the broken bone or bones, will in most cases give comfort. The strips should be an inch and a half wide, and six or eight inches long; they should overlap one another by one-third, run parallel with the ribs, and cover several sound ribs above and below the fracture.

Should the inflammation of the pleura or lung run high, it must be actively combated; the dressing being removed, and cupping, blistering, and general antiphlogistic measures resorted to. Under such circumstances, the fracture becomes a matter of secondary importance.

The same remarks apply to fractures of the costal cartilages.

Fractures of the Pelvis are only caused by tremendous violence, and are dangerous chiefly from the injury apt to be sustained by the viscera at the same time. If the urethra is ruptured, there will be blood trickling from the end of the penis; if the bladder is torn, there will be collapse, abdominal tenderness, and no discharge of urine per urethram. Rupture of the rectum is impossible from mere breaking of the bones, although a fragment has been known to pierce a portion of the small intestine.

When a fracture of the pelvis is suspected, the best plan is to proceed as if it were clearly made out; a broad roller should be firmly applied round the part, a few turns being taken round the upper part of each thigh to prevent the bandage from slipping upwards. The visceral injuries, if there be any, call for prompt and careful independent treatment.

§ 4.—FRACTURES OF THE BONES OF THE UPPER EXTREMITY.

Fractures of the Clavicle may be due either to direct blows, or to indirect violence, as in a fall on the hand

Fig. 67.

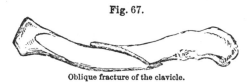

Oblique fracture of the clavicle.

or on the point of the shoulder. The bone is most apt to give way near the middle. Deformity always occurs,

Fig. 68.

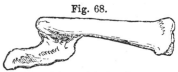

Fracture of the outer third of the clavicle.

the outer fragment usually slipping behind the inner, the pectoralis major and minor pulling the shoulder in-

Fig. 69.

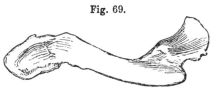

Fracture of the inner third of the clavicle.

ward and forward, while the weight of the upper extremity drags it down. The power of the arm and hand is always impaired, but to a degree varying with the amount of resolution to resist pain possessed by the

Fig. 70.

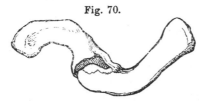

patient. Sometimes, especially after the first week or two, all the motions of the limb are perfect.

Compound fractures of this bone are extremely rare.

The indications for treatment are, to keep the shoulder upwards, outwards, and backwards. Reduction is generally easy, but its maintenance difficult. Various plans may be resorted to.

If a patient with a broken collar-bone could be kept perfectly still on his back in bed, union would occur without any deformity, at least in a large proportion of cases; and this position is therefore best even when an apparatus is used, although it is difficult to enforce it.

A simple posterior figure-of-8 of both shoulders has been recommended, but is irksome, and not always effectual. The same may be said of various forms of dressing on the same principle; the cruciform dorsal splints, the shoulders being fastened to the two ends of a transverse bar, the yoke splint, etc.

In many cases, a simple sling for the elbow, such as can be easily made with a large handkerchief, so arranged as to carry the elbow well across in front of the chest, and to raise it as much as possible, will meet the

13*

indications; at any rate, it is often the only available dressing for a time.

More complex forms of the sling have been contrived by Fox and Levis. Fox's apparatus consists of a sling to embrace the elbow, lower part of the arm, and nearly all the forearm; a stuffed ring or collar for the sound shoulder, and a wedge-shaped pad for the axilla. The pad and sling are fastened to the collar by tapes running across the chest in front and behind, and the hand is supported by a separate sling made of a strip of bandage or a handkerchief. (See *Fig.* 71.)

Fig. 71.

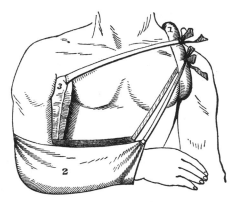

Fox's apparatus for fracture of the clavicle.—1. the collar; 2. the sling; 3. the pad.

Levis's apparatus consists of a pad for the axilla of the injured side, supported by tapes running up to be buckled at the top of the shoulder to a wide band, which runs thence around the back of the neck, and down in front of the sound shoulder, terminating in front of the corresponding axilla; close to this extremity it has buckled to it three tapes, two from the anterior corners of the sling, coming round the back, and one from its upper part at the back of the arm. (See *Fig.* 72.)

Fig. 72.

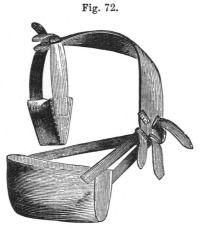

Levis's apparatus for fracture of the clavicle.

The plan described by M. Mayor* for the treatment of fracture of the clavicle will often be found more available than any other, especially as a temporary expedient. It requires a large handkerchief, or square piece of stuff, two bands or cravats, and in some cases a pad of cotton. The elbow being brought inwards, forwards, and upwards, so as to reduce the fracture, and the handkerchief folded into a triangle, the base of this triangle is applied to the front of the arm, and its ends carried round the body to be tied; the angles opposite the base hang down in front, and are now passed up behind the elbow and forearm. One of the supplement-

* Bandages et Appareils à Pansements; ou Nouveau Systéme de Déligation Chirurgicale. Paris, 1838.

ary bands is now attached to one of these single corners, the other to the other; one passes up on either side of the neck, and both then go down to be attached to the posterior portion of the triangle. The forearm and elbow are thus safely and firmly slung in the proper position. When the pad of cotton is employed, it is placed in the axilla of the injured side, and serves to render the bringing in of the elbow more efficient.

The foregoing are the principal modifications of the sling as applied to the treatment of fractured clavicle. Every case must, however, be treated for itself; the surgeon must not be satisfied, because he has put on an approved form of apparatus, that he has done everything, but must try to discover and meet all the indications that may be presented.

Desault's bandage for this injury has become obsolete; it is complex, uncomfortable, no more efficient and less easily watched than the dressings already mentioned. It consisted of three bandages and a long wedge-shaped pad; the first bandage kept the pad in place in the axilla; the second compressed the arm to the side, thus carrying the shoulder outwards; and the third, a figure-of-8 of three turns, pushed the shoulder upwards, outwards, and backwards.

Velpeau's bandage is much simpler, and when properly applied is very efficient; it is particularly suitable when the patient has to be transported some distance. A piece of linen or flannel rag being laid over the front of the chest, the hand of the injured side is brought up so as to rest upon the sound shoulder; a roller $2\frac{1}{2}$ inches in width is then applied, beginning in the sound axilla, passing across the back to the injured shoulder, down in front of the arm, under the elbow, up behind

and over the shoulder, and down across the front of the
chest to the original point of starting.   This having
been several times repeated, turns of the bandage are
made horizontally round the body and the arm of the
injured side, from below upward, until only the hand

Fig. 73.

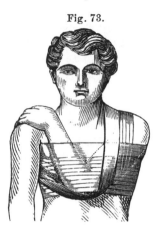

and the tip of the shoulder are left uncovered.   The
arm is thus bound to the trunk, the elbow being carried
inwards, forwards, and upwards, so as to force the
shoulder outwards, backwards, and upwards; and the
whole is secured by inserting pins wherever the turns
of the bandage cross one another.

Dr. David Gilbert, of this city, has described to the
author an apparatus used by him with great success in
fractures of the clavicle.   It consists of a pad for the
axilla, secured in place by the bight of an adhesive
strip 1½ inch wide and 3 feet long, the ends of which
cross one another over the sound shoulder; and of three
double adhesive strips, each 4 inches wide and 4½ feet

long. One of these surrounds the lower third of the arm and the body; the second is applied to the elbow, its ends being carried up to cross one another over the sound shoulder; the third passes round the elbow, the forearm, and the body. The hand is supported by a sling.

Fractures of *both* clavicles occur with extreme rarity, and are very difficult of treatment, mainly because the patients are so apt to object to the necessary restraint. Some modification of Velpeau's bandage, or of the old plan of Boyer,—with a brace buckled round the trunk and another round the arm, the two being fastened together,—or an arrangement of the starched or plaster bandage, will probably afford the best chance; but nonunion resulted in three of the six cases on record.*

Fig. 74.

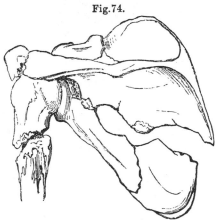

Fracture of the scapula and humerus.

Fractures of the Scapula are only caused by severe

---

* Malgaigne.

blows or by great crushing force; and they are always attended with great contusion. Hence the surgeon's first object must be to allay inflammation; this being accomplished, broad strips of adhesive plaster are first applied so as to form a cap for the shoulder, and then so as to confine the lower end of the scapula; the arm must be placed at perfect rest, by means of any convenient form of sling.

When the line of fracture runs through the neck of the bone and the base of the coracoid process, the surgeon should place a *small* wedge-shaped pad in the axilla, and put the upper extremity upon an inside angular splint, just as in fracture of the head of the humerus, to be presently described.

Fractures of the Humerus may be caused by any kind of force; by direct violence, by falls on the hand, or by muscular contraction, as in throwing a stone. The bone may be broken at any portion of its length; if close to either end, crepitus being perceived, the diagnosis often can be made out only by exclusion.

When the *head* of the bone is broken, a cap of pasteboard is fitted over the shoulder, or adhesive strips are applied so as to answer the same purpose. A flat splint is then applied along the inside of the arm, forearm, and hand, having an obtuse angle corresponding with the elbow, and another still more obtuse, with the wrist. The axillary end of this splint should be thickly padded. Permanent stiffening of the joint, in a greater or less degree, follows this injury; it is therefore best to use very careful passive motion after the third week.

Fig. 75.

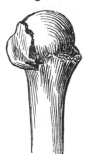

Fracture of the anatomical neck of the humerus.

Fracture of the *anatomical neck* (at the constriction just above the tuberosities) has very much the same symptoms but the line of division can be more clearly made out. The treatment called for is the same.

Fractures of the *surgical neck* of the humerus (between the anatomical neck and the insertion of the pectoralis major and latissimus dorsi) are somewhat difficult to treat; partly because of the disposition of the muscles to draw the lower fragments inwards, and partly because of the great leverage of the remainder of the limb, with the consequent risk of angular or rotary displacement. The diagnosis is usually easy.

The best plan of treatment is to put the limb upon an inside angular splint, like that for fracture of the upper end of the bone except in being most thickly padded at a lower point; a pasteboard, felt, or gutta-percha cap, fitted to the shoulder and upper three-fourths of the arm, being applied, and held in position by the upper turns of the bandage.—On an emergency, the arm may be placed akimbo over a pillow made into a pyramid, the apex of which corresponds to the elbow, and the base to the trunk; or a well-padded rectangular splint may be used in the same way.

Let it not be forgotten that the two points to be attended to are to support the humerus from the axilla to the elbow, and to keep the whole limb steady.

Fractures of the *shaft* of the humerus may be caused

either by direct or indirect violence. It is in this part that the bone gives way when broken by muscular contraction.

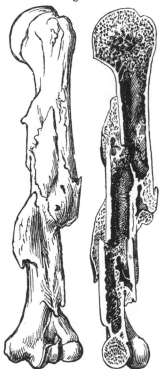

Fig. 76.

Absolute loss of power always occurs; and crepitus and abnormal mobility at the seat of injury indicate the nature of the lesion.

In some cases shortening of the arm is present.*

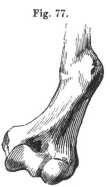

Fig. 77.

Fracture of humerus at lower third—showing deformity.

Splints are generally recognized as necessary in the treatment of these fractures. The best plan is to

Double fracture of the humerus.

use one long one, to steady the whole limb, and two or more short ones applied around the broken bone. The long splint, made either of wood or of very stout paste-

---

* The proper mode of measurement is from the tip of the acromion process above to the external condyle below.

board, should reach from well up in the axilla, along the inside of the arm and forearm, to the ends of the fingers; the elbow being bent at a right angle, and the hand semi-prone. The short splints should be three in number, and something less than two inches wide; the posterior one should be nearly as long as the back of the upper arm, the outer and anterior ones rather shorter than the distance from the axilla to the bend of the elbow. My objection to the anterior splint, as recommended by Amesbury, and still sometimes used, is that it cannot be so applied as to obtain as much purchase on the upper fragment as the inside one affords, and that it holds the hand in the supine position, which is less comfortable than the semiprone.

Or we may combine the anterior short splint with the inside angular one, by tacking a piece of pasteboard of the proper size and shape to the upper or arm portion

Fig. 78.

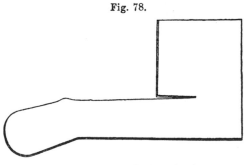

Angular splint made of pasteboard.

of the latter. When pasteboard is used, we may follow the outline of the inside angular splint, but make the upper portion, above the angle, a little more than twice the usual width; and then, cutting a slit half way across it, continuous with the upper edge of the forearm part, we have a portion which may be bent over so as to fit the front of the arm.

It is easy to see how the same purpose might be answered with a piece of stout wire, bent so as to form a frame for the limb, well wrapped in bandage, and secured like any other splint.

When long splints are for the time unattainable, Boyer's plan may be resorted to; it consists in applying two or three short splints around the arm, and then, the axilla being well padded, confining the whole limb to the body with a bandage. However carefully carried out, this plan would be apt not to prevent displacement of the fragments, the apparatus becoming deranged by the movements of the patient.

Shortening, if marked, must be obviated by the use of an inside splint, with a well-padded head going far up into the axilla; or by putting along the back or outside of the arm a special splint, long enough to allow of extending bands being carried from its upper end beneath the axilla and from its lower end round the bend of the elbow.

In compound fractures of the arm, where bone is lost to any extent, there is danger of lengthening, so that the fragments will always remain separated by an interval, and the member be rendered nearly or quite useless. This lengthening may be due to the mere weight of the lower part of the limb, but it may be caused also by injudicious splinting. Caution on this point should always be observed.

Fracture of the *lower portion* of the humerus, whether the joint be implicated or not, is apt to prove troublesome.

Crepitus is sometimes the only distinct evidence of the nature of this injury, and the diagnosis of its seat and direction can only be made out by exclusion, especially when the swelling is great. The line followed by the fracture varies much in different cases.

Fig. 79.

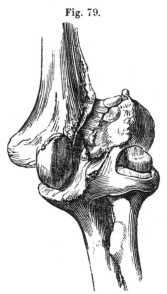

Fracture of outer condyle of humerus.

Fig. 80.

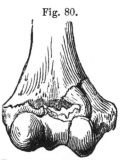

Fracture of humerus just above the condyles.

So much swelling and inflammation occur in fractures near the elbow, that the surgeon generally has at first to make free use of local antiphlogistics and anodynes,—leeches, lead-water alone or combined with laudanum, or ice-water; the patient being placed in bed, and the limb laid easily on a pillow. Purging and diaphoresis may also be called for. As soon as the inflammation and tenderness have subsided, the arm may be flexed at a right angle, and bound to a well-padded anterior splint. After four or five days the right-angled splint may be exchanged for one with an obtuse angle; and in two or three days this again may be replaced by an acute-

angled one. By some surgeons, a single splint with a
changeable angle regulated by Stromeyer's screw, is
preferred; but the angle should never be altered to any
marked degree without removing the splint from the

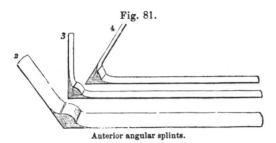

Fig. 81.

Anterior angular splints.

limb. A frame of strong wire, bent to the desired
angle, wrapped in bandage, has been used as a substitute for the angular wooden splint with advantage by
army surgeons.

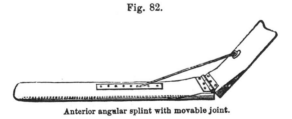

Fig. 82.

Anterior angular splint with movable joint.

When both the upper and lower bones constituting
the elbow-joint are broken, when the inflammation and
swelling have run high, and when passive motion is very
painful, the surgeon will do better to keep the elbow
flexed at a right angle, so that if anchylosis should
ensue the limb may not be rendered wholly useless, as it
would be in the straight position.

14*

Fracture of the *olecranon process of the ulna* is rare.
It has mostly been observed as the result of direct violence, but there are on record several authentic instances
of it from muscular contraction.   The signs of this injury are inability on the part of the patient to straighten
the arm, pain, swelling, and more or less perceptible
separation of the fragments, the triceps muscle drawing
the upper one away from the lower.   Crepitus will
sometimes, for an obvious reason, be wanting.

Fig. 83.

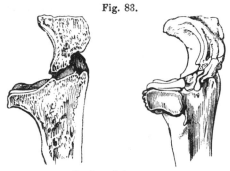

Fracture of olecranon.

The treatment consists in placing the arm in the straight
position, and fixing the upper fragment against the lower
by means of strips of adhesive plaster applied semi-
elliptically above it.   In order to keep the arm extended, it should be bound to a straight anterior splint
reaching from a point opposite the axilla to the roots of
the fingers; gradually the extension may be relaxed,
as the fragments become united.*   Union is almost cer-

* Having successfully employed the hooks for fracture of the
patella, invented by M. Malgaigne, I have thought that an analogous
instrument might be devised for the olecranon; but have as yet had
no opportunity of carrying out the idea.

tain to be ligamentous, so that the arm fails to regain its strength; and some stiffening of the joint is extremely apt to ensue.

Fractures of the *bones of the forearm*, below the elbow, are by no means uncommon. Both bones may be crushed at any point; indirect force may cause them to give way either at the same or at different points in their length, but always somewhere near the middle. When indirect force breaks only one of them, it is the radius which gives way at or near its lower extremity.

Fig. 84.

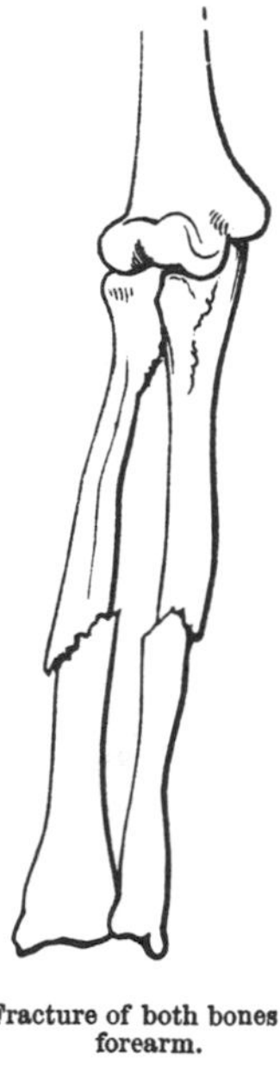

(1) If both bones are broken. By reference to the articulated skeleton it will readily be seen that the radius and ulna are exactly on a plane with one another only when the thumb is upward, and also that the interosseous space is greatest in this position. And by mechanical laws it may be shown that the ease and power of pronation and supination, the most important movements of the hand, depend on the maintenance of this space. Hence in all cases of fracture of the forearm, the proper rule is to keep the hand semiprone.

Fracture of both bones of forearm.

Pain, loss of power, deformity, abnormal mobility, and crepitation, are the reliable symptoms of an injury of this kind. Two splints should be applied, one on the anterior and the other on the posterior face of the forearm; the former extending from the elbow to the fingers, the latter about as long as the radius. The former may be shaped to the outline of the forearm and

Fig. 85.

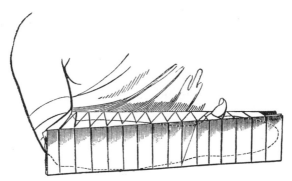

Double splint for fracture of both bones of forearm.

palm, with a block at the lower end to be grasped in the fingers; the angle at the wrist, causing abduction of

Fig. 86.

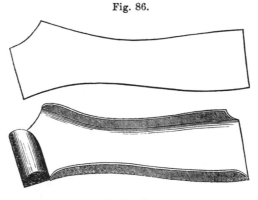

Bond's splint.

the hand, is important when the fragments of the radius show any tendency to overlap one another: Both splints being padded, the padding being thicker along the centre, so as to press into the interosseous space, are applied, and retained by means either of a roller or of broad strips of adhesive plaster.

Should the patient be from any cause likely to move the hand from the semiprone position, the anterior splint should be extended up the inside of the upper arm, constituting an inside angular splint; this will effectually prevent any rotation of the fragments. The application of a bandage directly to the forearm can do no possible good in these cases, and may do much harm.

(2) If one bone is broken, be it the radius or the ulna, at any portion of its shaft, the same treatment as in the last case is proper.

The *radius* may be fractured by muscular action, as I saw in one case, when it had yielded at its neck while the patient was pulling very hard in driving. But it is far more commonly broken at or near its lower extremity, by indirect violence, as in falls on the hand.

Fig. 87.

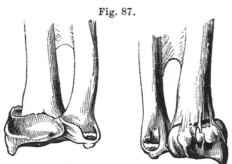

Colles's fracture of the radius.

The line of division may run transversely, an inch or so above the joint end of the bone; or the styloid pro-

cess of the radius may be broken off, the fracture running obliquely downward into the joint.   In the former
case, we speak of it as Colles's fracture, Dr. Colles, of
Dublin, having first accurately described it;* the latter

Fig. 88.

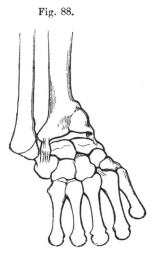

Barton's fracture of the radius.

is called Barton's fracture, attention having been called
to it by Dr. John Rhea Barton, of this city.†

Whichever of these injuries may be present, the symptoms are almost the same; there is swelling at the back
of the wrist, some sinking in at the corresponding
point in front, total loss of power in the hand, and pain
on pressure or passive motion.

The treatment differs slightly in the twó cases; extension of the broken bone, by drawing the hand over

---

* Edinburgh Med. and Surg. Journal, April, 1814.
† Am. Journal of the Med. Sciences, 1840.

towards the ulnar side, being much more necessary in the oblique than in the transverse fracture. One splint, such as is known as Bond's, shaped to correspond to the outline of the forearm and hand, with a block so placed as to be grasped in the hand, (a firm pad of cotton or

Fig. 89.

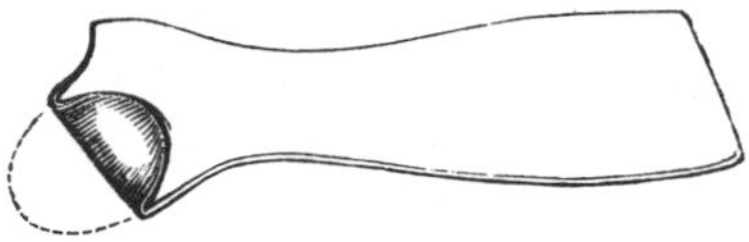

Bond's splint as made of pasteboard.

any other suitable or convenient material may be substituted,) is necessary. When strong pasteboard is used, it may be cut into such a shape that the end, being rolled over, will answer the same purpose as the block. This being duly covered, the arm is bound to it with a roller. When the prominence at the back of the wrist tends to recur, another posterior splint thould be added, with a compress so disposed as to make the required pressure.

Although there may be no impairment of either strength or motion left on recovery from these fractures, deformity is very apt to remain—a fact of which the patient should be forewarned.

Fractures of the *carpal* bones are always due to direct violence, and may be followed by necrosis. Perfect rest, with a dozen leeches, if they can be had, should be first applied, and antiphlogistic and anodyne lotions (iced lead-water is the best) should be used for several days; and then, the rest having been strictly maintained for a week longer, passive motion may be very cautiously attempted.

The *metacarpal* bones may be broken by a crushing force; or a man strikes a blow with his fist, and one end

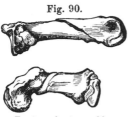

Fig. 90.

Fracture of metacarpal bones.

of a metacarpal bone impinges upon a resisting part, such as the edge of the orbit, when the bone yields at some portion of its length. Usually the lesion is recognized without difficulty. The treatment consists in fixing the hand by binding a ball or thick pad in its grasp.

Bond's splint (*Figs.* 86 and 89) answers the purpose very well.

Fractures of the *phalanges* may be treated best by placing the hand in a hemispherical block of soft wood, with grooves cut in it so that the fingers may rest comfortably in them; or if plaster of Paris can be had, by mixing a little, letting it nearly set, and then causing the patient to put his hand on it, pressing the fingers down so as to form grooves. By means of adhesive plaster or a roller, the injured bone may be kept accurately in place. Passive motion should be resorted to in the course of the second week.

It sometimes happens that two or more fractures occur at once in the upper extremity; the one furthest from the trunk has then to be first attended to. Thus I have several times seen the upper part of the humerus and the lower part of the forearm broken in the same limb. These cases simply call for an adaptation of the ordinary methods of treatment, by splints of a mixed form; the surgeon can often make such out of heavy binder's-board.

§ 5.—FRACTURES OF THE BONES OF THE LOWER EXTREMITIES.

It is almost impossible for the femur or tibia to be broken without the patient being rendered incapable of walking or even standing; if he can manage to crawl along, it is apt to be with great pain and difficulty, while all such efforts involve the risk of subsequent inflammation, deformity and perhaps loss of life. In the case of any bone or bones of the tarsus or metatarsus, or of the phalanges, although standing or walking is out of the question, the less leverage upon the fragments will allow of the patient dragging himself along on all fours after a fashion. But in all these injuries the rule is imperative that the surgeon should place the part as soon and as completely at rest as possible. Hence the matter of *transportation* becomes of great moment, as accidents of this kind seldom happen first at the spot where the treatment is to be carried on. Especially in military surgery, where the cases are most severe, and the circumstances most trying, is this subject important.

The chief rules for transportation have been already laid down in speaking of the general subject of fractures; but some special points call for notice here. It may be well to repeat that carrying by hand is far better than any other plan; and that a four-wheeled wagon is better than a cart. For obvious reasons, water transport, when available, is greatly to be preferred to that by land.

As the fragments are disturbed by any motion whatever of the head or trunk, the patient should be directed or compelled to lie perfectly still on his back.

15

One of the best and simplest means of confining a fractured lower extremity can almost always be had; it is only strange that it should be so little known. This is to take a bundle of straw, the stiffer the better, (wheat-straw is the best,) and to enclose the limb in it, the component straws lying parallel to the axis of the limb. Hay, the stems of bushes, corn-stalks or leaves, twigs, or small sticks may be substituted if suitable straw cannot be had. The limb and its envelope may now be bound round with wisps of straw, strings, or bandages of any kind, care being taken not to compress the seat of fracture too tightly. Greater firmness may be given by inserting two or more sticks among the straws at either side of the limb. Should swelling now occur, the dressing will yield, the straws being simply drawn out in the direction of their length. The state of the part may be readily watched; hæmorrhage will be at once manifest; and in order to modify or remove the dressing, we have only to loosen the circular bands. Extension and counter-extension may be made in various ways upon a limb thus drawn up, if needful.

A box on the plan of the *fracture-box*, to be hereafter described, may be readily knocked together in a few minutes when the necessary boards and tools can be had; and stuffed with straw, will serve to keep the limb properly secured even for a journey of some length.

Let it never be forgotten, when a patient with fracture has to be sent any distance without medical supervision, that the worst danger is from circular constriction; even motion of the fragments involves less risk than this.

Extension and counter-extension are often desirable during the transportation, either to prevent shortening of the limb, or to keep it steady. With a view to this it is best to pass any convenient band under the back, bringing its ends up by way of the axillæ and in front of the shoulders, to be fastened either to pegs driven in the floor of the wagon, or to the upper cross-piece of the stretcher if one is used. Another band, looped in a figure-of-8 on the dorsum of the foot and under the tendo-Achillis, and secured in like manner by its ends to a peg or to the lower cross-piece of the stretcher, will serve to make extension. A less effective plan some-times has to be resorted to,—passing the counter-extend-ing band over the perineum, and tying it to the upper end of a board or stick, to the lower end of which the extend-ing band is fastened. In either method the bands may be applied without removing the patient's clothing.

When time permits, and a few boards can be had, a very good plan is to have a box knocked together, con-sisting of a bottom and two sides. The outer side should be long enough to reach from 4 inches below the foot to the axilla, or at least above the crista ilii, the inner one from the same point to the perineum; the bottom, smoothly bevelled off above at its upper end, should reach from the tuber ischii as far down as the other two. Counter-extension may be made from the perineum as in the ordinary Physick's Desault's apparatus, to be presently described, extension by any convenient band fastened to a peg driven either across between the two sides, which is best, or vertically into the bottom of the box near its lower end. Straw, hay, sand, bran, cot-ton, tow, or even leaves, may be used to embed the limb and prevent its contact with the wood.

Fracture-bed.—Whenever patients have to be strictly confined to bed, lying on the back, as in the injuries now to be considered, it is obvious that some provision must be made for the removal of discharges from the bowels and bladder. Bed-pans and urinals of different kinds are to be found in the shops, but (the former at

Fig. 91.

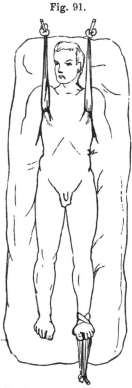

Extension and counter-extension, as made in transporting patients with fractures of the lower extremity.

Fig. 92.

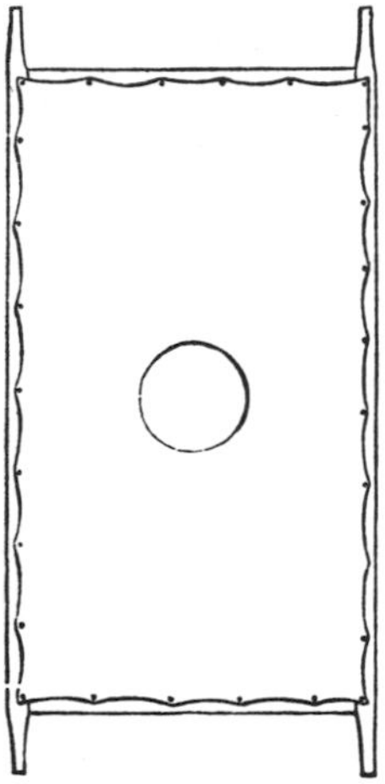

Sacking-bottom frame for fracture-bed.

least) involve too much moving of the patient in their use. Hence it is customary to arrange the bed so that the same end may be better answered. One plan is to have a strong sacking-bottom, with a hole cut at the centre, set in a frame of the same size as the mattress, upon which it is laid; hinged under the frame are four legs eight or ten inches long. This, with the patient on it, can be raised up, set on the legs, and a chamber introduced under it; the bowels being relieved, the chamber is taken away, and the sacking-bottom is let down again on the mattress. Another plan is merely to have an opening cut in the mattress, with a pad to fill it up when it is not needed. Two cleets nailed across beneath the bedstead-frame serve to support the chamber, the rim of which slides along them. Various other forms of fracture-bed have been devised, but need not be described here.

Bed-sores.—These may be properly spoken of here, because they are apt to occur in old, weakly or heavy persons, during the long confinement to bed rendered necessary by fractures of the lower limbs. They should be carefully guarded against by changes of posture; by frequent bathing of points pressed upon, as the sacrum and hips, with stimulating liniments, common rye whiskey being as good as anything else for the purpose; by protecting such parts with soap plaster spread on kid; and when circumstances permit, by the use of air-pillows or flat India-rubber bags partly filled with water.

FRACTURES OF THE FEMUR.—As would be judged *a priori* from the shape of this bone, it may be broken at one or more of many points. By far the largest number of cases, however, occur within the middle third of its length, in man; in women the upper third of the bone gives way more frequently in proportion. The neck of the femur may be broken, by indirect violence,

15*

applied either over the trochanter or at the lower end of
the bone; the fracture is *intra-* or *extra-capsular*, ac-

Fig. 93.

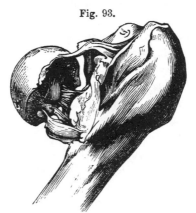

Intra-capsular fracture of femur.

cording as it does or does not affect the bone above the
annular attachment of the capsule of the hip-joint.

Fig. 94.

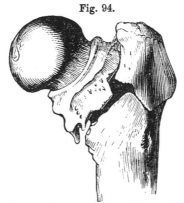

Fracture of neck of femur (extra-capsular) with fracture of great trochanter.

When it runs obliquely, so as to enter the joint only at
one portion of its extent, the two forms are combined.

The greater trochanter may be detached by direct force. The shaft of the femur may give way near the intertrochanteric line, usually as the result of indirect vio-

Fig. 95. Fig. 96.

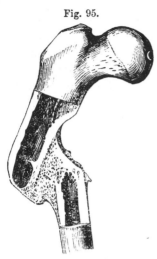

Fracture of upper third of femur. Fracture of lower third of femur.

lence; in a few cases on record, muscular action has caused this fracture. In the middle third of the shaft, fractures may be produced by any form of violence; the line of division is apt to be markedly oblique. At the lower third we may have either a fracture through the lower part of the diaphysis, a separation of the epiphysis, or a breakage running not only across the bone but down into the joint; so that there are three fragments. Or one condyle may be broken off by itself.

The *diagnosis* of fractures of the femur is in general easy, except when the bone is broken very high up, close to or within the joint, when there may be much doubt as to whether the injury is a fracture or a luxation.

The symptoms common to both forms of injury are shortening,* pain, difficulty or loss of motion of the joint, persistent eversion or inversion of the foot. But in fracture the shortening, which may usually be overcome by traction, returns again as soon as the limb is left to itself; while in luxation it does not recur if once corrected. In fracture the foot may be rotated by the surgeon, while in luxation this can be done only to a very small extent, if at all. In fracture crepitus can be elicited, in luxation none. Fracture is much more likely to be present if the patient is old, while dislocation is more common in the young.

Still, there are cases of this kind which baffle the utmost care and attention of the surgeon, and a decision should never be hastily arrived at.

It is sometimes a matter of great importance to accurately determine the amount of shortening present. The pelvis being placed on an exact plane, and the limbs at equal angles with its transverse axis, the measuring tape should be carried from the anterior superior spine to the edge of the inner malleolus, passing to the inner side of the patella. The limb supposed to be shortened should be measured first.

The *treatment* of fractures of the thigh is a subject of the highest importance.

When the bone is broken within the capsule of the hip-joint, the surgeon should warn the patient and his friends that a complete cure can scarcely be looked for, since bony union seldom if ever takes place.

In very old persons, the best plan is simply to place

---

* The luxation downwards and forwards, with lengthening of the limb, is so rare and so easily recognized that it needs no exceptional mention in the text.

them in bed and keep them as comfortable as possible; guarding against inflammation of the joint, and preventing the occurrence of bed-sores. Sometimes the capsular ligament becomes so thickened as to enable the patient to walk tolerably well, with the aid of a crutch or cane.

Younger persons may be similarly treated, except that it is worth while to use a pasteboard splint moulded to the hip and thigh, in order to retain the joint at perfect rest. Bony union is declared by some writers to have occurred even in intra-capsular fractures. When there exists a strong tendency to shortening, extension and counter extension should be made by fastening the shoulders and the foot of the injured side to the head and foot of the bed respectively.

Fractures of the great trochanter are very rare. The fragment is drawn upward and backward by the glutæi muscles, and the power of eversion of the limb is greatly impaired.

Adhesive strips, applied as in fracture of the olecranon, should be employed to bear the broken piece down into its position; and a compress and bandage over them may add to their efficiency.* The limb should be confined by means of a pasteboard splint, as in the last-mentioned case.

Fractures just below the trochanters are apt to be troublesome from the tilting up of the upper fragment by the action of the psoas magnus and iliacus internus

---

* I would suggest here also the idea of employing steel points to catch the upper edge of the fragment, on the principle of Malgaigne's patella-hooks; a band around the upper part of the thigh giving them a *point d'appui.*

muscles.   More or less shortening and deformity, with
permanent lameness, are apt to ensue in these cases.
It being impossible, for want of purchase for pressure,
to bring the upper fragment down, we have to resort
to the expedient of bringing the lower fragment up,
by means of a double inclined plane. (See *Fig*. 102.)
After about three weeks have elapsed, the knee may be
gradually lowered, in the hope that the new material
may be strong enough to maintain the relation of the
fragments.   A pasteboard splint carefully moulded and
secured to the front of the thigh will add to the safety
of this procedure.

Fractures of the middle third of the femur are apt to
be followed by more or less shortening of the limb, due
to overlapping of the fragments.   Hence the patient
will ever afterwards limp, unless he wears a high-heeled
shoe; there is very seldom any loss of power.

For no other injury have so many methods of treatment been proposed as for this; and perhaps in none is
an altogether satisfactory result more infrequent.   We
have already spoken of the surgeon's duty in regard to
the transportation of his patient, and shall now describe
the plans available for the subsequent management of
the case.

The methods employed at the present day may all be
divided into two classes, according as they are or are not
based on the principle of extension; the former are the
most numerous, and the most generally to be relied upon.

A very simple and excellent plan, when the patient
is not very restless and uncontrollable, consists in fastening the shoulders to the head of the bed by means of
a folded towel or other band passing round the back and

up in front of the shoulders by way of the axillæ; extension is now made by hanging a weight, attached to the foot, over the foot of the bed. From 5 to 30 pounds will be required, according to the age and degree of muscular development of the patient.

Dr. Gurdon Buck of New York uses an apparatus on this principle, but makes his counter-extension from the perineum to the head of the bed, while he introduces a piece of gum-elastic in the extending band. He employs also four "coaptation-splints," to surround the thigh, lying parallel with it; maintaining them in place by means of three elastic bands with buckles.

Another form of these splints, used by the late Dr. Horner of Philadelphia, is shown in *Fig.* 97. The con-

Fig. 97.

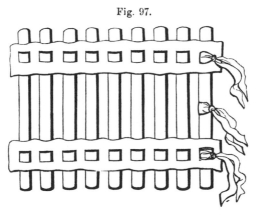

Horner's coaptation-splints.

necting bands may be readily made of muslin, flannel or leather; gum-elastic is better when it can be had. Perhaps it need hardly be remarked that the splints should never be placed in immediate contact with the skin.

But the best apparatus for treating fracture of the

thigh by extension, when surrounding circumstances are favorable, is based upon Desault's plan as modified by Physick. It consists of two splints of thin board, one reaching from near the axilla to a point a few inches beyond the sole, the other from the perineum to just below the inner malleolus. Near the upper end of the long or outside splint are cut two holes for the attachment of the counter-extending band; the means of making the extension and counter-extension are so various as to call for separate notice presently. Between each splint and the limb is of course an irregular interval; these are filled up either by long muslin bags stuffed with hair or bran, (junk-bags,) or, what is better, with pieces of old flannel folded in three or four thicknesses. In order to give stability to the apparatus, it has been, and still is with many surgeons, customary to use a splint-cloth, or piece of muslin as wide as the length of the inside splint wrapped around both splints; and the whole is tied with three strips of bandage passing transversely. But the splint-cloth is useless, the same purpose being served by giving each of the circular strips of bandage a turn round each splint, enclosing also the lining, which is thus kept in place; either of these may be tightened or loosened without destroying the rest. The circular strips will be sure to stretch somewhat during the first 24 or 48 hours; after that they may be made more secure by tacking them to the edges of the splints. A

Fig. 98.

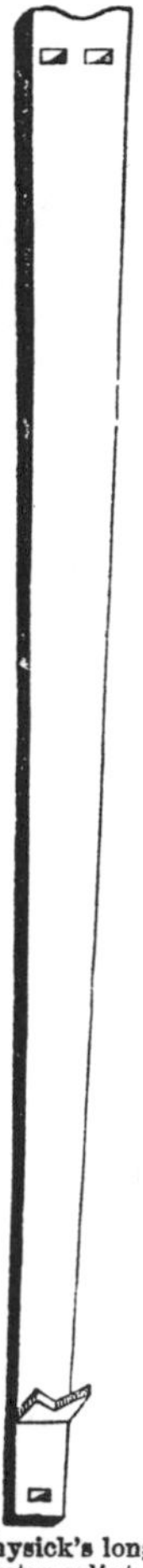

Physick's long outer splint.

broader strip is used in the same way to keep the splint and the pelvis together, and still another should confine the trunk to the splint near its upper end.

Counter-extension may be made by means of a tube of buckskin or muslin, stuffed with hair or bran, with tapes at its extremities to pass through the holes in the outside splint and to be tied at its upper end. This is known as Coates' perineal band; if the perineum is daily washed with whiskey, *and carefully dried before the band is reapplied*, there is little or no danger of excoriation.—On an emergency, any band may be used as a temporary substitute; a skein of yarn answers extremely well.— Another method, chiefly advocated by Dr. D. Gilbert of Philadelphia, is by means of adhesive plaster. He uses "double anterior and posterior strips about four inches wide, crossing each other over the trochanter of the *sound* side, and passing over the pelvis diagonally, anteriorly and posteriorly, to a little above the crest of the ilium on the side of the

Fig. 99.

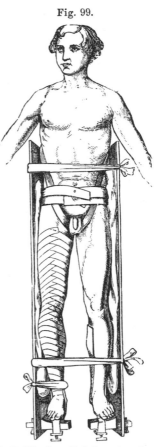

Dr. D. Gilbert's method of counter-extension by adhesive plaster.

fracture; then crossing each other again, and passing through holes in the upper part of the splint to be tied firmly on its outside. The splint is more nearly Desault's in length, commanding the movements of the pelvis and entire lower extremity, and converting them as it were into *one solid piece for the time being.*"* (See *Fig.* 99.)

Extension may be temporarily made by means of a handkerchief or a strip of bandage tied in a figure-of-8 around the dorsum of the foot and back of the heel. But by far the best method is with adhesive plaster, as follows: A strip 2 inches wide, and twice as long as from the seat of fracture to three inches below the sole of the foot, is stretched as much as possible. A bit of thin wood, 4 inches in length by 3 in width, is next fitted to the middle of its adhesive surface, and on either side of this a slit is cut lengthwise in the plaster. Through these two slits a strip of bandage is now passed, so that the bit of wood is between the bandage

Fig. 100.

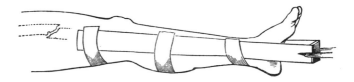

Extension by adhesive plaster in fractures of the thigh.

and the adhesive strip. The two ends of the adhesive strips being now applied up along each side of the

* In a note to the author, Nov., 1862. Dr. Gilbert's published papers may be found in the *Am. Journal of Med. Sciences* for Jan., 1851, Jan., 1858, and Jan., 1859.

limb, with the block of wood 2 inches from the sole of the foot, will just about reach the seat of fracture. It is a matter of importance that the thin piece of wood just mentioned should be so wide as to take off the pressure of the extending bands where it passes over the malleoli; its long diameter (4 inches in the case of an adult male) should correspond to the length of the strip. Three circular strips should be applied, one above and one below the knee, and one just above the ankle, to keep the longitudinal one in place; they should not entirely surround the limb, lest the return of venous blood be impeded. It will now be found that strong extension may be made by pulling on the two ends of the bandage. These are carried over a block placed on the inner side of the long splint, about four inches below the sole; one passes round the end of the splint, and the other through a hole just above it, so that they meet to be tied together. — When circumstances permit, it is an excellent plan to arrange a horizontal pulley at the lower end of the outer splint, and to let the extending

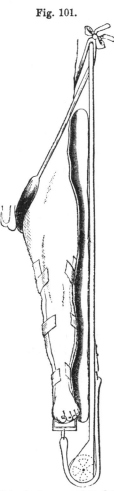

Fig. 101.

Extension by means of an elastic band, as employed by the author.

band play over this; the band itself, or a portion of it, being made of a strong India-rubber cord or loop, and fastened at the outside of the splint. (*Fig.* 101.) In this way we allow for spasm of the muscles, and at the same time keep up an unremitting tension on the limb.*
—One objection holds against all the various forms of screw-arrangements for tightening the extending band; it is that they are no more efficient than other means against the real difficulties of the case, which are: the tenderness of the skin, rendering it unable to bear pressure, and the yielding of the bands employed. At the same time, the power so easily exerted with the screw may cause great suffering to the patient.

The various forms of the inclined plane act on the principle of extension and counter-extension, but less efficiently than those already described; the weight of the body is the counter-extending force in most of them. The single inclined plane is made by fastening together two boards, one vertical and the other inclined towards it at any suitable angle; the inclined one should be a few inches longer than the lower extremities of the patient, and should join the other a little below its upper end. The patient lying on his back, with the fractured limb placed on the inclined plane and fastened to the vertical board, the weight of the body will be continually drawing down the upper fragment; the surface on which the limb rests should of course be padded.

The double inclined plane is much more complex. It consists of two boards, fastened together at an angle to fit that of the knee; the foot is supported and steadied

---

* See a paper on this subject by the author, in the *Am. Journal* for July, 1862.

by another piece of board corresponding to its sole.
Usually sides are added to each portion, either nailed on
or hinged; and the leg and thigh-pieces are also hinged
together, being kept at any desired angle by means of
a rackwork.

Fig. 102.

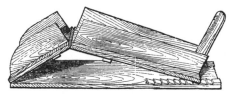

Double inclined plane.

It is evident that in this machine the counter-extension
is made by the weight of the body, the extension by the
pressure of the upper part of the leg-piece against the corresponding part of the limb. But here, as in the single
inclined plane, the tendency will be for the patient to
work along up the inclined surface with his buttocks, so
as to defeat the intention of the surgeon.

A new form of the inclined plane, which has gained
much favor, has not long since been introduced by Dr.
N. R. Smith of Baltimore. It consists of a rectangular
frame of stout iron wire, about 3 inches wide at one end,
and $2\frac{1}{2}$ or $2\frac{3}{4}$ at the other; it is intended to reach from a
little above the spine of the ilium to a point just beyond
the toes, and should therefore be about 3 feet 8 inches
long for a man of ordinary stature. Cross-pieces of wire
are firmly clinched to the side-pieces at intervals of
about 8 inches. There are also two double hooks of
wire, each of which is adapted to clip the side wires
firmly, and has a loop above like a figure-of-8, forming
an eye for the attachment of a suspending cord. A small

16*

pulley and a tent-block are useful, but not indispensable to the apparatus. When the splint is to be applied, it is bent so as to correspond with the front of the limb

Fig. 103.

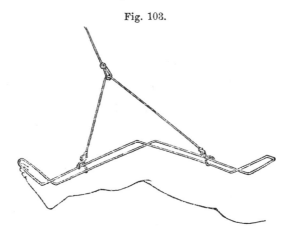

Diagram showing the principle of Dr. N. R. Smith's anterior wire-splint for fracture of the thigh.

when the hip, knee, and ankle are somewhat flexed; it is then wrapped in the turns of a bandage, and the limb bound to its under surface. The double hooks are now made to catch the splint at about the middle of the thigh and leg, and a cord attached to both; to the middle of this cord is tied the end of another, rove through the tent-block and passing over the pulley, which is fastened to the ceiling. Extension is made in proportion to the degree of slant assumed by this latter cord when the limb is thus suspended; the weight of the body is the counter-extending force. If the extension is not made properly, or if the splint presses too much or too little above or below, the points of the attachment of the sus-pending cord should be changed; and the efficiency of the apparatus may be enhanced by raising the foot of the bed with blocks.

The simplicity and efficiency of this splint have led to its extensive use in army practice in this country. It may be rendered still more secure by adding a starched or dextrinated bandage to the one which immediately surrounds the splint and limb.*

At a late stage of the treatment, when union has duly taken place, and the callus simply needs support, some form of the immovable apparatus may be found useful. Thus a starched bandage carefully applied about the fourth or fifth week will enable the patient to get out of bed, and to move about a little with crutches.

Fractures of *both* thighs should be treated in the same way as when only one limb is injured. If the patient is a child, or a restless and unmanageable adult, an anterior splint of pasteboard should be applied to each thigh at about the tenth day; the long splints should be extended up into the axilla, and furnished with crutch-heads, while a cross-bar should be arranged between them at the lower ends.

Fractures of the patella are not very common. When vertical or longitudinal (the rarest form) they are always due to direct violence, and are chiefly serious on account of the inflammation likely to be set up in the joint. The treatment has reference wholly to this dangerous sequence.

---

* A splint on the same principle, and made in like manner of iron wire, may be found described and figured in Mayor's "Nouveau Systéme de Déligation Chirurgicale," published in Paris in 1838. Mayor's splint, however, was intended to go beneath the limb, which rested upon it.

Transverse fractures of the patella may be caused by force directly applied, such as a blow; or the bone may

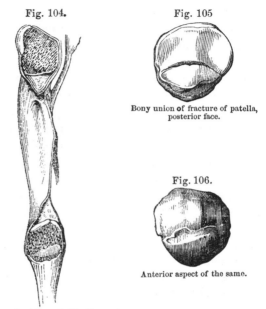

Fig. 104.

Fig. 105

Bony union of fracture of patella, posterior face.

Fig. 106.

Anterior aspect of the same.

Fracture of patella united by ligament.

be broken by muscular contraction, being bent as a lever over the lower anterior edge of the femur.   More or less separation of the fragments immediately takes place, and persists or even increases afterwards; on account of the difficulty of overcoming this, union is apt to be ligamentous only.

As a matter of course, the muscles should first be relaxed by straightening the limb, and flexing the thigh on the trunk, and then the upper fragment should be drawn down into the closest possible proximity to the

lower.   Various plans have been proposed for retaining
it thus.   The plan most simple and available is that of
Dr. Sanborn of Lowell, Mass.   A strip of adhesive
plaster about two feet long is laid on the anterior surface of the leg and thigh, about six inches being lifted

Fig. 107.

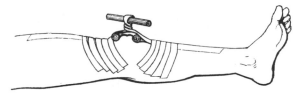

Sanborn's plan of securing fragments of patella.

up into a loop in front of the knee.   A bandage is now
firmly applied from the toes up, leaving the loop of
course free.   The upper fragment being now drawn
down as much as possible, a firm transverse compress is
laid just above it, and the loop twisted by means of a
bit of stick so as to bear upon the fragment through the
compress.   A posterior splint completes the apparatus.
Malgaigne's hooks—a pair of steel plates sliding upon
one another, and recurved at their extremities into two
opposing pair of sharp hooks, intended to catch the
upper and lower edges of the fragments, the hooks being
forced together by a screw playing longitudinally above
the plates,—are more formidable in appearance than in
reality.*   I can decidedly recommend their use, from
experience.—Adhesive strips may be applied in a cres-
centic form above the upper fragment; or, as recom-

---

* See a report of a case in which they were twice used, by the
author, in the *Am. Journal*, April, 1861.

mended by Sir A. Cooper, longitudinal tapes may be arranged along the sides of the knee, and circular bandages above and below; the latter being then drawn together by turning over the end of the former and tying them.—Lonsdale's instrument is complicated and expensive.

FRACTURES OF THE BONES OF THE LEG are extremely common, and may be caused by any form of external violence. The diagnosis is usually a matter of no difficulty. Shortening is not often present in any marked degree, but sometimes demands special attention.

Fig. 108.

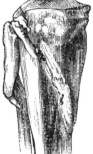

Fracture of upper end of tibia and fibula.

It is in these cases that the *fracture-box* has been most extensively used. This consists of a bottom, two sides hinged or nailed to it, and a foot-piece fastened vertically or nearly so ; the latter projecting up above the level of the toes. A pillow laid in the box gives equable support to the limb, and the foot is steadied by fastening it to the foot-board.

Fig. 109.

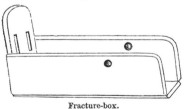

Fracture-box.

Counter-extension may be made from the sides of the box, by adhesive plaster, if necessary.

By a little mechanical ingenuity the fracture-box may be so suspended to a stout frame placed in the bed as

Fig. 110.

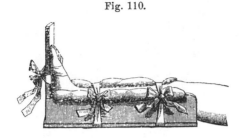

Fracture-box applied.

to enable the patient to move in bed somewhat without disturbing the fragments in their relation to one another; and the tedium of his confinement will thus be greatly lessened.

Some surgeons employ lateral splints of pasteboard, kept in place either by broad strips of adhesive plaster or by a roller; if the latter, it should commence at the toes.

When *both bones are broken low down*, there is usually what is called "Pott's fracture;" the fibula yielding about three inches above the joint, and the inner malleolus, or the whole lower extremity of the tibia, being also separated. If the fibula alone is broken, with rupture of the internal lateral ligament of the ankle, the deformity and other symptoms will be much the same.

The treatment consists in placing the foot in a fracture-box, and using applications to allay inflammation of the joint, for about two weeks; at the end of that

Fig. 111.

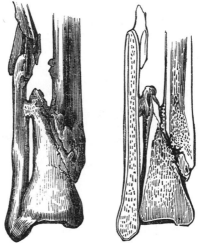

Fracture of tibia and fibula at lower part.

time Dupuytren's apparatus should be put on;—a splint three or four inches wide, extending from the knee three inches beyond the sole of the foot, with a thick wedge-

Fig. 112.

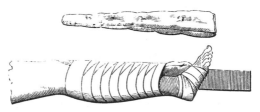

Dupuytren's pad and splint applied.

shaped pad whose base is placed just above the malleo-lus, bound firmly to the inner side of the leg.   No attempt at walking should be made by the patient for at least six weeks. — The jointed splint of Dr. N. R. Smith of Baltimore answers extremely well for the treatment of these fractures of the leg low down. Its modus operandi may be best understood by examining it; it is kept for sale by most instrument-makers.

Fig. 113.

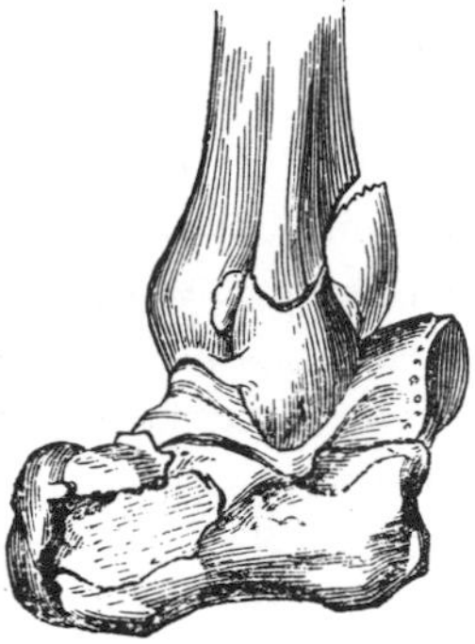

Fracture of the *os calcis* may be caused by the weight of the body, suddenly and violently brought to bear upon the heel.

Fracture of calcaneum and lower end of fibula.

It can hardly fail to be recognized; the treatment consists in extending the foot as much as possible, bringing down the fragment by means of adhesive strips, and placing a pasteboard splint along the front of the leg and dorsum of the foot. A roller firmly applied from the toes upward completes the dressing.

Fig. 114.

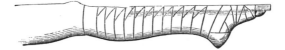

Fractures of the *metatarsal* and *phalangeal* bones, when not attended with such injury of the soft parts as to require amputation, are usually recognized mainly by the crepitus on handling. The swelling soon masks even this. Negative treatment only is necessary; when union

17

is nearly complete, a firmly applied bandage will enable the patient to make cautious attempts at walking.

¿ 6.—COMPOUND FRACTURES.

It is in injuries of this class that the question of amputation, resection, or conservation most frequently comes up. With this point we have now nothing to do. When it is decided that the saving of the limb may be properly attempted, the surgeon's great aim should be to close the wound which, by forming a communication between the break in the bone and the atmosphere, constitutes the injury a compound fracture; or in other words to render the compound fracture a simple one.

Keeping this in mind, the case is to be dealt with on general principles. Dry lint or cotton may be employed to close the wound if it is small; the limb being subsequently splinted and bandaged as in the case of a simple fracture. If the skin and subjacent tissues are extensively lacerated, the edges of the rent must be brought together with isinglass or adhesive plaster, or with compresses and a bandage.

Should one or both of the fragments project through the wound, so as to be irreducible, and prevent its closure, they should be sawn off; and any loose pieces of bone should be extracted.

Swelling must always be provided for; it is so sure to occur as to forbid the use of sutures except in rare cases.

As far as possible, the surgeon should content himself with simply supporting the injured limb; but the manner in which this is done must vary with the bone involved. Sometimes the limb will do best laid on a pillow, with a cold or warm water-dressing over the wound; ice-water, when it can be had, will often be found to give great comfort, especially during the first few days. If there is any tendency to displacement, or if the patient is restless, the arm may be lightly fastened on a splint, or the lower extremity confined by means of a fracture-box or Desault's apparatus. Sand-bags—made like the ordinary junk-bags already described, except that sand is used to stuff them instead of bran—may be laid along on either side of the lower extremity, if it is the thigh or leg that is injured; and extension, when called for, may be best made by means of adhesive plaster, with a weight hanging over the lower end of the bed. Often the fracture-box may be adapted to the upper extremity with advantage.

In hot weather, Barton's *bran-dressing* — the limb being laid on a bed of dry bran in a fracture-box, and surrounded and covered with the same material—will prove a valuable resource. Extension and counter-extension may of course be readily made at the same time, if desirable.

Whatever plan of treatment is adopted in these cases, it is of importance to attend to the constitutional condition of the patient. During the first few days, fever will be apt to occur, and must be subdued by low diet, cooling drinks, and the avoidance of noise or excitement. Bleeding is seldom if ever called for, and has the disadvantage of lowering the patient's power of resistance, which will be needed for the subsequent task of recovery. Purgatives must be sparingly used, as their action involves more or less motion on the part of the patient, and the fracture is thus disturbed.

§ 7.—NON-UNION, PSEUDARTHROSIS, OR FALSE-JOINT.

Usually the degree of motion, which for a fortnight or more is plainly perceptible at the seat of a fracture, becomes less and less until consolidation of the fragments is effected. When this access of firmness takes place very slowly, we speak of the case as one of *delayed* union; but no special treatment is called for, except to improve the patient's general health.

In other cases, the ends of the fragments become rounded off, and remain wholly unconnected with one another. Again, they may be fastened together more or less loosely by bands of fibrous tissue.—Or, lastly, within the mass of fibrous tissue, and between the broken ends, there may be formed a sort of bursa, strongly resembling the synovial sac of a regular joint.

This condition of things may depend either upon the state of the patient's general health, or upon some local cause, such as the interposition of a bit of muscle or a splinter of bone between the fragments, inefficient dressings, etc.

Many plans have been proposed for inducing union in these cases. The first thing to be done is to remove all impediments, as far as we can; to improve the constitutional condition; and to keep the parts at absolute rest for two or three weeks by careful splinting. Should the degree of mobility now seem lessened, we may persevere for six or eight weeks longer in the same course.

Should the progress made during this time be unsatisfactory, we may rub the fragments smartly together until pain is caused, and then place them again at rest for several weeks. This failing, if it is the lower extremity that is affected, we may put the broken bone up in moulded splints, supporting it well, and let the patient walk about.   Dr. H. H. Smith of this city has contrived a special apparatus, something like the "irons" used to

Fig. 115.

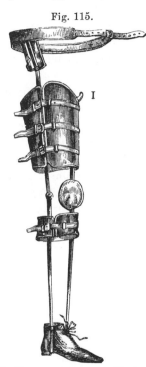

I

Smith's apparatus for ununited fracture of the thigh.

Fig. 116.

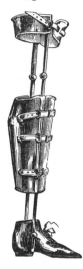

Smith's apparatus for ununited fracture of the leg.

correct bow-legs in children, to act as an artificial support in these cases.*

Electro-puncture, according to rules elsewhere laid down, may next be tried.

---

* *Am. Journal of the Med. Sciences,* Jan., 1855.   See also Smith's *Practice of Surgery.*

We may now employ Brainard's plan of boring the ends of the bone in two or three points with an awl, introduced through the skin.   Dieffenbach drove small ivory pegs into the awl-holes.

The bone remaining still ununited, we may resort to Physick's plan of passing a seton through the limb, between the fragments; avoiding of course the large vessels and nerves.

Or, in patients whose constitutional state is suitable, we may expose the broken ends, saw or rasp them off, and place them in apposition.   Some surgeons have cauterized the fractured ends thus exposed, and others have wired them together; the latter measure seems more promising than the former.   Such operations, however, are among the most serious known to surgery, and should never be lightly undertaken; it would be foreign to the scope of this book to describe them in detail.

CHAPTER VIII.

DISLOCATIONS.

By *dislocation* or *luxation* of a bone, is meant the escape of its articulating extremity nearest the trunk from the corresponding surface. Thus the humerus is said to be dislocated when its head leaves the glenoid cavity of the scapula. The ball-and socket joints are those most subject to luxation.

Dislocations may be caused by a direct force knocking the head of the bone into its false position, or by violence acting upon the distal end, the whole bone forming a lever by means of which its head is displaced. They are in all cases either *simple* or *compound*, and either of these may be *complicated;* these terms having the same significance as when used with reference to fractures. When the head of the bone has wholly left the corresponding surface, the luxation is said to be *complete;* when it still remains partly in contact with it, *incomplete* or *partial.* The luxation is said to be *primitive* when the head of the bone retains the false position it first assumes, *consecutive* when it has undergone a further change of place. The terms *recent* and *old* would seem to need no explanation; but they are conventionally applied to luxations before and after the lapse of about a month. They are in some measure arbitrary.

Pain, deformity, and impairment of motion are the chief and most constant symptoms of this class of in-

juries; sometimes the limb is shortened, and much more
rarely lengthened. In cases of doubtful diagnosis between fracture and dislocation, the probabilities are in
favor of the former if the patient is either very young
or very old, or a female, more evenly balanced if a male
in middle life. Whenever the nature of the injury is
obscure, the surgeon may derive great assistance, and
the patient be saved much pain, if the latter is made insensible by means of ether or chloroform before the examination is begun.

The luxated head of a bone must return to its normal
position, if at all, by the same course as that by which
it escaped. Often the capsular ligament has sustained
a rent like a button-hole, and the most enormous force
would be unavailing to replace the head of the bone
unless applied in the proper direction. Hence, in order
to an understanding of the indications in any case, the
surgeon must be fully acquainted with the anatomy of
the joint concerned, as well as of the soft parts surrounding it, and must inquire with diligence into the
exact mode in which the displacement has been induced.

Until within a few years past, it was thought by surgeons that powerful extension was called for in almost
every luxation, although in the case of the hip, as Hamilton remarks, "reduction by manipulation dates from
the earliest records of our science." This process of
reduction by manipulation is now employed in displacements of nearly all the joints, and will perhaps altogether supersede, in recent cases, the old method with
its formidable array of pulleys and assistants. Perhaps
it need hardly be said that the surgeon should always
make trial of manipulation before resorting to other
measures. The general rule seems to be recognized

that the muscles should be as much as possible relaxed, and the limb moved in the direction in which the least resistance is encountered. A clear understanding of the points already referred to will of course enable the surgeon to proceed more methodically, and with a better prospect of success, than if he merely moves the limb in different directions in the hope of hitting the right one.

Reduction should invariably be attempted at the earliest possible moment. Before the introduction of anæsthesia by ether or chloroform, surgeons were accustomed to abolish muscular resistance by bleeding their patients to faintness, by the warm bath, by tartarized antimony, by tobacco, or by alcoholic intoxication; these latter means are now of course done away with.

§ 1.—LUXATIONS OF THE LOWER JAW.

Both condyles of the lower jaw may be displaced in front of the glenoid cavities, by a force which greatly depresses the bone at its symphysis, such as a downward blow when the mouth is open ; the accident may also be caused, in weakly persons, by the act of yawning widely. This is *complete* luxation. (See *Fig.* 117.)

Incomplete or *partial* luxation occurs when only one condyle is thus displaced; it is much rarer than the first form, but has the same mechanism.

When both condyles are out, the mouth is fixed wide open ; a depression exists in front of the lower part of the external ear; the patient is unable to speak, and cannot swallow, so that the saliva accumulates and flows away; sometimes there is also much crampy pain, especially in the temporal muscles. When only one condyle is luxated, the jaw is twisted to the other side, and brought slightly forward; the mouth is slightly open; the depression and pain are on the injured side only.

Fig. 117.

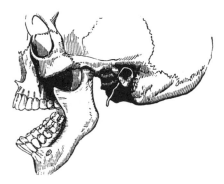

Complete luxation of the jaw.

It is evident that in order to replace the jaw, the condyles must be depressed below the level of the anterior margins of the glenoid cavities. This may be done in several ways. The best plan is for the surgeon, standing in front of his patient, who is seated on a low, firm chair, or on the floor, to elevate the symphysis of the jaw with his fingers, while he bears down on the molars of each side with his thumbs, well wrapped to avoid being bitten as the jaw snaps into its place. Some surgeons put a cork or pad over the molars, to serve, like the thumbs, as a fulcrum, the jaw-bone being acted on as a lever of the first order. Or the surgeon may stand behind his patient, and employ the same mechanism, supporting the head against his own chest. Or one side may be restored first, and then the other; the partial luxation being dealt with on the same principle as the complete. A supporting bandage should be used for a week or two.

In old or enfeebled patients especially, this manipulation may sometimes be successfully employed without putting the thumbs inside the mouth, pressure being made downward against the cheeks; such a case occurred to me quite recently in an old colored woman.

A subluxation of both condyles forward may be simulated by a spasmodic contraction of the depressing muscles of the jaw. It yields gradually to anodyne frictions and fomentations.

¿ 2.—DISLOCATIONS OF THE VERTEBRÆ.

These injuries, unattended with fracture, are very rare; they are more apt to affect the cervical region than the dorsal or lumbar. They owe their importance to the danger they involve to the spinal marrow.

Cases of this kind are upon record in which surgical interference has proved successful; extension and rotation being carefully made until the displacement was overcome. Perfect rest for weeks afterward is advisable.

¿ 3.—DISLOCATIONS OF THE RIBS.

Although a rib may possibly be displaced from its posterior connection, a detachment of its anterior end from the cartilage is much oftener met with. Several ribs may be thus luxated, without any danger being necessarily involved. The signs and treatment are obvious.

¿ 4.—DISLOCATIONS OF THE CLAVICLE.

Either end of the clavicle may be luxated. The sternal end may be driven backward by a direct blow, when the large vessels at the root of the neck will of course be endangered. Or, as has oftener happened, an indirect force throws the end of the clavicle in front of the sternum, or upward along the side of the trachea. The diagnosis in such cases can hardly be difficult. Reduction should be effected by manipulation, the shoulder being drawn outwards and downwards or upwards as the case may require. An apparatus much like that for fracture of the clavicle, modified to suit the case, should be employed to keep the bone in place when reduced. Complete restoration of the parts can seldom if ever be permanently effected; but the use of the arm may be very little impaired.

The acromial end of the clavicle may be displaced upwards, so as to rest on the upper surface of the acromion process. Such an accident may generally be recognized on careful examination. Reduction is not difficult, but the bone tends to slip out again very readily; hence in addition to a sling confining the arm, direct pressure by a compress and strap is requisite.

A very few cases are on record in which the acromial end of the clavicle is said to have been dislocated downwards; in all, reduction was effected and maintained with ease.

§ 5.—DISLOCATIONS OF THE SHOULDER.

The humerus may be displaced from the glenoid cavity of the scapula *downwards, forwards* or *backwards.*

(1) *Dislocation downwards.*—This may be due either to direct or to indirect force. On examination, there will be found a depression below the acromion; the head

of the humerus forms a lump in the axilla; the elbow is carried out some inches from the body, and more or less rigidly fixed; the arm slightly lengthened, and the whole limb somewhat numb from pressure on the axillary nerves. It will be found impossible to carry the hand of the injured side across to the sound shoulder.

When recent, a luxation of this kind is usually reduced without much trouble, chloroform or ether being always given unless contraindicated. The patient is seated on the ground or on a firm chair; the surgeon faces him, kneeling or standing before the injured shoulder, and puts his nearest knee in the axilla, under the displaced bone, while he bears down with his corresponding hand upon the shoulder, so as to fix the scapula. Now, keeping his leg vertical, he grasps with his free hand the lower part of the dislocated arm, and by means of it swings the patient up over his knee, the outer edge of which constitutes a fulcrum over which the humerus bears as a lever of the first order. Generally, after a few trials, or it may be at the first, the head of the bone goes in with a snap. Should the surgeon be short-legged or the patient long-bodied, it will be necessary to place a firm block under the foot of the former. Here the principle is the same as in the old plan of swinging the patient up by his arm over the edge of a door or the round of a ladder.—Another plan is to bind one loop of a roller towel firmly to the lower end of the arm with a wet bandage ; the patient then lying down, the surgeon sits so as to place his heel* in the axilla, the free loop of the towel being cast over his back and one shoulder; he now grasps the wrist with one hand and the forearm

---

* His boot of course being first removed.

high up with the other, so as to rotate the arm by using the forearm as a lever, and makes extension by bearing backward with his body and straightening his hip and knee-joints. The force is begun and increased gradually, so as not to stimulate the muscles to resistance; having been strongly kept up for a few moments, it is suddenly relaxed. An assistant should steady the scapula by pressure from above.—Some surgeons, among whom is Mr. Skey of London, employ the pulleys for extension, while a roller or other hard body is placed in the axilla, and counter-extension is made from a staple fixed in the wall.—Another plan, proposed by Dr. N. R. Smith of Baltimore, is to seat the patient on a firm chair, a little on one side of it, so as to allow room on the side of the injury for the operator's foot; a long piece of stout muslin is then passed around the chest, under the injured axilla, and its tails carried horizontally, in front and behind, to be secured to the wall or some other unyielding point; to this band the wrist of the extended

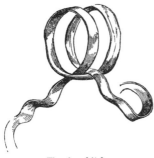

Fig. 118.

The clove-hitch.

sound arm is firmly bandaged. An ordinary roller is carried back and forth over the injured shoulder and under the muslin band, twice, and then three or four times around under the seat of the chair and over the shoulder. A wet roller being applied to the wrist of the injured side, the extending band is then fastened to it by means of the clove-hitch, and traction made by two persons, outward and at first somewhat downward, then horizontally, and then a little upward, the force being gradually increased. Should this not succeed, the surgeon places his knee under the head of the bone, while the traction is made upward as much as possible; this having been done for a few moments, the arm is suddenly brought downward.—Another and a very old method is to sweep the elbow by steady force outward and upward until the arm is parallel with the neck, making traction all the while; the patient lying on his back, and the surgeon sitting so as to operate with one hand while he steadies the scapula with the other. If more strength is needed, the surgeon may apply his foot on the top of the shoulder, while he operates with both hands; or he may employ assistants.

Dr. H. H. Smith, of Philadelphia, claims* to have devised the following method of reducing these luxations, by rotation and elevation of the humerus: "In the anterior luxation, elevate the elbow as much as possible, and carry it toward the head of the patient, keeping the arm on the line of the body, when the head of the humerus will readily slip into the axilla. In a posterior luxation, elevate the elbow, and carry it forward so as to free the head of the humerus from the edge of the scapula, so as to throw it into the axilla, as has been long practised. An anterior or posterior luxation may also be readily converted into an axillary or subglenoid, by elevating the elbow and carrying it backward—the capsular ligament in each luxation being freely lacerated by the injury.

"The head of the bone being now mainly held against

* Smith's Surgery, vol. i. p. 720.

the neck of the scapula by the contracted supra and infra-spinatus, proceed as follows:—

"Elevate the elbow and arm as high as possible, and flex the forearm at right angles with the arm, thus relaxing the supra-spinatus muscle. Then, using the forearm as a lever, rotate the head of the humerus upward and forward, so as to relax the infra-spinatus, carrying the rotation as far as possible, or until resisted by the action of the subscapularis muscle, keeping the forearm for a few seconds in its position with the palm of the hand looking upward; then bring the elbow promptly but steadily down to the side, carrying the elbow towards the body, and keeping the forearm so that the palm of the hand yet looks to the surgeon. Then quickly but gently rotate the head of the humerus upward and outward by carrying the palm of the hand downward and across the patient's body, and the bone will usually be replaced."

(2) *Dislocation forwards* may be either primitive, or consecutive upon dislocation downwards; the only important difference between the two being, that in the former case the rent in the capsule will be in front, and in the latter below. Sometimes the head of the bone lies just below the coracoid process, sometimes higher up, just under the clavicle. The elbow is directed slightly backwards, and the arm very slightly shortened, if changed at all in length.

Reduction is effected by analogous means to those used in luxation downwards, but the operation would seem to be less generally successful than in that case.

(3) *Dislocation backwards* is rare. It has been ob-

served as the result of direct violence in some cases, of indirect in others. It has generally been recognized without any particular trouble, and reduced by much the same methods as the luxation downwards.

In any of these cases, after the bone has been replaced, the arm should be confined for at least ten days or two weeks in a sling, inflammation of the joint being prevented by the use of antiphlogistics generally and locally. A recurrence of the accident is always likely to happen.

Old Dislocations of the shoulder have always been regarded as troublesome and even dangerous to meddle with. After the lapse of six or eight weeks, the head of the humerus becomes more or less bound in its false position by adhesions, as well as by stiffening and contraction of the muscles. Very great force is almost always requisite to overcome these obstacles to reduction, and sometimes the attempt has to be abandoned. Moreover, it should not be forgotten that not only has the bone sometimes been broken, but cases are upon record in which fatal rupture of the axillary artery has taken place; so that very great caution is necessary in undertaking and performing the operation.

Besides the other mechanical means already mentioned, there is an instrument known as "Jarvis's adjuster," too complicated to be described here, which may be used with advantage in breaking up the adhesions, so that the bone may be reduced in the ordinary way.

¿ 6.—DISLOCATIONS OF THE ELBOW.

BOTH BONES of the elbow may be dislocated *backwards*, the fibres of the brachialis anticus muscle being usually torn, or the coronoid process of the ulna broken off. The joint is almost rigid, bent at an obtuse angle, its antero-posterior diameter much increased; the olecranon projects backwards much as the os calcis does at the heel.

Fig. 119.

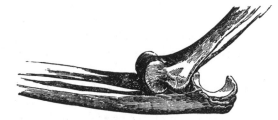

To reduce this luxation, the forearm must be drawn downwards until the coronoid process of the ulna clears the posterior edge of the articulating surface of the humerus, when the normal form of the joint is at once restored, and flexion to a right angle becomes possible. An inside angular splint should be used to support the arm for a week or two, and if necessary, inflammation should be combated.

BOTH BONES of the forearm may be dislocated *forwards*, either with or without fracture of the olecranon;* but this accident is much rarer than the preceding. The symptoms are shortening of the arm and lengthening of the forearm, absence of the olecranon at its usual place, tension of the skin, and slight flexion of the elbow. The elbow may be straightened, or even bent forwards; but only with great pain.

---

* See Am. Journal of the Med. Sciences, July, 1862, p. 248; also Hamilton on Fractures and Dislocations, p. 594.

Reduction is easily effected by strongly flexing the elbow, over the arm of an assistant if necessary.

When the radius and ulna are luxated *outwards*, the elbow is bent somewhat, and the head of the radius can be felt outside of the articulating extremity of the humerus; the hand is pronated. The diagnosis is not difficult.

Reduction is generally easy in recent cases, the surgeon placing his knee in the bend of the elbow, while with one hand he grasps the upper arm, and with the other draws down and attempts to flex the forearm upon it. Should this prove painful, or fail, simple extension with assistants, while the surgeon makes lateral pressure, may succeed.

Luxation of these bones *inwards* resembles the last-mentioned case, except in the deformity about the joint, the bony points being different. The treatment is to be conducted on analogous principles.

The ULNA alone may be dislocated backwards, but there is usually at the same time a fracture of the outer condyle of the humerus. Its treatment should be like that of luxation of both bones backwards, an anterior angular splint being applied afterwards.

The RADIUS alone may be dislocated *forwards, backwards, or outwards,* the latter being thought by Hamilton to be usually consecutive upon either one of the former. The annular ligament must of course be either stretched or torn in these cases; it is generally torn. Sometimes the luxation *forwards* is irreducible; and it is always, like both the other forms, very apt to recur. The treatment consists in manipulation and direct pressure.

§ 7.—DISLOCATIONS OF THE WRIST.

The wrist may be luxated either *backwards* or *forwards*, the latter being the less common form.   I have once seen all the carpal bones displaced into the palm of the hand, by crushing between two calico-rollers; they were restored by manipulation, but the subsequent inflammation caused the loss of the hand.

In luxation backwards, there is a prominence at the back of the wrist, and another in front, the latter being nearer the ends of the fingers than the former.

Fig. 120.

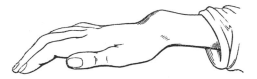

Dislocation forward of the wrist.

In luxation forwards, the prominence at the back of the wrist is on a line with the back of the forearm, and nearer the ends of the fingers than in front.   In both, the motions of the joint are lost, and the hand rendered useless.

The treatment consists in making extension on the hand, rocking it back and forward so as to make the convexity of the carpus clear the edge of the concave articulating surface of the radius.   Having thus restored the bones to their proper relation, an anterior and posterior splint, with suitable compresses, should be applied. Inflammation should be carefully subdued.

Sometimes, especially in weakly and loose-jointed persons, the os magnum is started out of place so as to form a prominence at the back of the hand; the displacement is usually permanent, and when it can be corrected is apt to recur.

§ 8.—DISLOCATIONS OF THE METACARPAL BONES.

The metacarpal bone of the *thumb* may be dislocated either towards the dorsal or palmar surface of the trapezium; the injury can be readily recognized and treated.

Very rarely indeed, the other metacarpal bones may be displaced backwards. Hamilton* mentions having seen two cases of this luxation of the index and middle fingers; in both, the lesion was caused by striking a blow with the clenched fist, and had proved incurable.

§ 9.—DISLOCATIONS OF THE PHALANGES.

Of all these bones, the first phalanx of the thumb is most frequently luxated, and generally backwards. Sometimes it stands erect upon its base, near the lower end

Fig. 121.

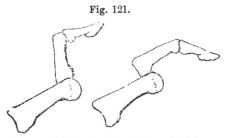

Diagram of dislocation of first phalanx of thumb.

of the posterior surface of the metacarpal bone; sometimes it has assumed a direction nearly parallel to the latter.

---

* Op. cit., p. 607.

Mere extension will often fail in the reduction of this displacement; it may be tried, a piece of strong tape being attached to the thumb, just above the last joint, in a clove-hitch.

Failing in this, the surgeon should try manipulation, on the plan suggested by Dr. Batchelder of New York.* With one hand Dr. B. recommends flexing the metacarpal bone as much as possible into the palm of the hand, so as to relax the flexor brevis pollicis; then pushing forward the upper end of the dislocated phalanx, the surgeon, grasping its distal end, makes forcible flexion and extension. After proceeding thus for a few moments, he suddenly flexes the thumb strongly; if it is not reduced, he bears the distal end back again so as to bring the phalanx at a right angle with the metacarpal bone, (still keeping up the pressure against the upper extremity of the former,) when the luxated bone will slip into its proper place.

Such manipulations may be very properly combined with extension. In order to obtain a firmer hold of the luxated phalanx, various methods have been devised; Charriére, the well-known French instrument-maker, has made a forceps for the purpose. But the simplest plan is that of Dr. Levis of this city, with a slip of hard wood perforated with holes, through which tapes are passed so as to form two loops; the dislocated thumb or finger being embraced between these loops and the wood, the loops are drawn tight and secured so by winding the tapes around the upper end of the bit of wood.

For mere extension, the Indian " puzzle," a tube of

---

* New York Journal of Medicine, May, 1856.

braided straw, which narrows as it is pulled upon, answers very well; the finger is introduced into it, and it cannot let go until the traction is relaxed.

Division of the lateral ligaments (of the tendons of the flexor brevis in the case of the thumb) has been proposed and executed by many surgeons, and may be resorted to with propriety if all other means fail.

§ 10.—DISLOCATIONS OF THE HIP.

It is of the utmost importance for the surgeon to recognize and treat properly these very serious injuries.

Fig. 122.   Fig. 123.

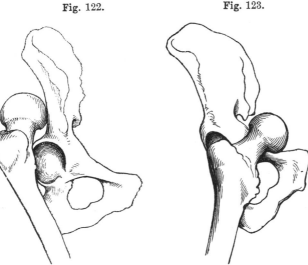

Dislocation of the head of the femur upon the dorsum ilii.

Dislocation of the head of the femur forward upon the pubis.

Four general forms of them are described, although cases occur in which the head of the femur assumes some intermediate position. It may be displaced:

(1) *Upwards and backwards* upon the dorsum ilii.

(2) *Backwards* into the sciatic notch.

(3) *Upwards and forwards* upon the pubis.

(4) *Downwards and forwards* into the foramen thyroideum.

Fig. 124.

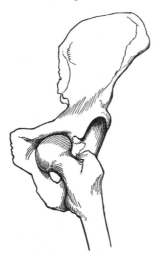

Dislocation of the head of the femur into the foramen thyroideum.

In the first form, the limb is much shortened, and the toe inverted; the thigh is adducted and somewhat flexed, so that the knee rests just above the patella of the opposite side; the trochanter major is nearer the anterior superior spinous process of the ilium than it should be, and the head of the femur forms an abnormal prominence. The buttock is widened and flattened.

In the second form, the symptoms are much the same as in the first, but less pronounced, and the head of the bone can be felt lower down, while the trochanter is carried only slightly upwards.

In the third form, the symptoms are quite different; the thigh is abducted and slightly flexed, the limb shortened, and the trochanter rendered obscure, while the head of the bone forms a marked prominence at the fold of the groin.

In the fourth form, the thigh is lengthened and somewhat adducted, the body drawn forwards towards it, the hip flattened, and a hollow felt where the trochanter should be.

Other directions in which the head of the thigh-bone has been known to be displaced are: directly upwards, directly downwards, downwards and backwards either into the lower sciatic notch, or upon the body of the ischium.

In any case of luxation at the hip-joint, the surgeon should first try to reduce by manipulation alone.   The mode of doing this will vary of course with the direction of the displacement, but the general rule is to bring the limb up towards the body, adducting, abducting and rotating it, so as in the first place to relax the muscles, and in the second place to cause the head of the femur to clear the lip of the acetabulum.   " Reid's method " of reducing luxations of the femur upon the dorsum ilii may be taken as a type of these procedures generally; it consists in flexing the knee, carrying it inwards across that of the sound side, and then sweeping it round up over the umbilicus and into abduction, rotating it at the same time.   Any one may arrive at the rationale of this proceeding, by going through with it a few times with a pelvis and an articulated leg, bearing in mind the while the exact anatomy of the soft parts about the joint; and the mode of dealing with the other displacements of the hip may be studied in like manner.   These movements should never be forced, but the surgeon should try a new direction as soon as he meets with any obstacle; he has perfect command of the limb in the leverage afforded

19

him by the thigh and leg.* Anæsthetics are hardly called for in this operation unless the patient is very timid, or an unusual degree of muscular spasm is present.

Mere manipulation failing, the surgeon must combine extension with it. Counter-extension is made from the perineum, extension from the lower part of the thigh; the counter-extending band being usually a sheet folded cravatwise, and attached to a staple conveniently fixed, while the extending force is made by assistants, either with or without pulleys.

The simplest mode of applying the extending force is by a strong band applied in a clove-hitch over a wet roller bound round firmly just above the knee. The ends of this band may either be knotted and attached to a set of pulleys, or arranged to be drawn upon by assistants. A leather band buckled round the thigh, having at right angles to it two straps terminating in rings, is sometimes used, but offers no advantages over the simple clove-hitch. Sometimes it is desirable to fix the body of the patient; and this may be done by means either of a broad belt or girth of webbing, buckled round the body, or by tying a folded sheet around the body and bedstead or table.

Occasionally traction has to be made in still another direction, at right angles to the axis of the bone, by means of a band carried round the upper part of the thigh, so as to draw the head of the bone outwards.

All being made ready, the patient being rendered wholly insensible by ether or chloroform, the surgeon

---

* For the fuller discussion and description of the various manipulations adapted to special forms of this displacement, the reader is referred to the treatises of Sir A. Cooper, Malgaigne, and Hamilton.

takes the leg in both hands, and while the assistants make the extension, rotates the thigh; or, committing this duty to a reliable assistant, he endeavors by direct pressure with his fingers to push the head of the femur into place.*

Reduction being effected, the thighs should be brought close together, and fastened thus by a bandage; the patient should keep his bed for at least a week.

A few words only need be said with regard to the remaining dislocations of the lower extremity.

§ 11.—DISLOCATIONS OF THE PATELLA.

A blow may knock the patella out of place, either outwards or inwards, or may twist it on its vertical axis.

No difficulty can exist in regard to the diagnosis, but the replacement of the bone may be a matter of impossibility. The patient being placed fully under the influence of an anæsthetic, the limb should be straightened as completely as possible, and the surgeon should then endeavor with his fingers to push the bone into its normal position. Failing in this, he should divide subcutaneously the fibrous structures which hinder the reduction, cutting if necessary even the ligamentum patellæ. The limb should then be placed absolutely at rest, and every means taken to prevent or allay inflammation.

§ 12.—DISLOCATIONS OF THE TIBIA.

By a direct blow, the tibia may be luxated upon the

---

* A correct knowledge of the anatomy of the hip will enable the student to apply the principles now laid down to any case of dislocation of that joint; while without such knowledge the minutest directions for each special form would prove useless.

femur either outwards, inwards, forwards or backwards; or the same result may ensue from the foot being firmly fixed in any way, while the body, with the thigh, is forcibly moved. In the first or second form of displacement, the bones are only partly separated, the inner condyle of the femur resting upon the outer articular surface of the tibia in the dislocation inwards, and *vice versâ*. In the third or fourth, the axes of the two bones may be quite parallel, and their articulating surfaces wholly removed from one another; the ligaments about the joint are more or less extensively torn, and the connections of the patella are apt to be broken either above or below; the popliteal vessels and nerve are endangered.

Neither the diagnosis nor the indications for treatment are obscure in these cases. Extension and counter-extension should be made by assistants, while the surgeon manipulates the bone into its place; and then the danger of inflammation is to be met. Amputation will be called for if the vessels and nerves have been broken across.

§ 13.—DISLOCATIONS OF THE FIBULA.

The upper end of the fibula may be displaced either forwards or backwards; the nature of the injury can hardly escape detection, and its treatment is very simple. It may be combined with a fracture of the tibia lower down.

§ 14.—DISLOCATIONS OF THE ANKLE.

By falls on the feet, or in railroad or machinery accidents, the ankle may be dislocated in various ways. The astragalus, with the calcaneum and other bones, may be carried backwards, or more rarely forwards, with regard to the lower end of the tibia and fibula. The astragalus alone may be dislocated, usually by violent wrenching of the foot; it may be felt forming an unnatural prominence in its new position.

Often the violence to the soft parts is so great, even when these luxations are not compound, as to cause destructive inflammation of the foot. The surgeon should however attempt reduction as early as possible, by means of extension and counter-extension made with the hands, the foot being at the same time flexed, extended, and moved in various directions, while direct pressure is exerted to force the bone into place.

Excision of the bone has been performed, where reduction was impossible, but without encouraging results.

¿ 15.—DISLOCATIONS OF THE SMALLER BONES OF THE FOOT.

These, when recognized, may sometimes be corrected without any great difficulty, by direct pressure. The surgeon should deal with them on the same principle as with those of the corresponding bones of the hand.

¿ 16.—COMPOUND DISLOCATIONS.

These are among the most formidable injuries met with by the surgeon. When it is possible, they should be reduced, and the attempt made, as in compound fractures, to render them simple by closing the wound. The subject is, however, beyond the province of Minor Surgery.

19*

CHAPTER IX.

CATHETERIZATION.

(THE term catheterization, being derived from the Greek verb *Καθιημι, I explore*, might properly include a very wide range of operations; but custom has limited it almost entirely to the introduction of instruments into the urethra. It is, however, with the curious inconsistency of our language, extended so as to embrace all the other instruments, as well as those which are strictly exploratory; while the word catheter, again, signifies only a tube for drawing off the urine or for injecting other liquids.

We shall speak first of the introduction of instruments into the urethra, and then of the other rarer and less important catheterizations.)

The instruments introduced through the urethra are of different kinds, according to the objects in view.

Catheters may be of metal or of gum-elastic; the metal generally used is silver, more or less alloyed.

Formerly, catheters were made with a very large curve, and something of an *f* shape. At present they are only curved for a short distance near the end; a healthy urethra would admit of their introduction even if perfectly straight. The modern shape is much better, because the surgeon can more readily tell exactly where the point of the instrument is as it passes along the deeper portions of the canal. Gum-elastic catheters are

(218)

of course destitute of fixed curve, and therefore stiffness is given them by means of iron wire introduced along their calibre, whenever they are to be used.

Eyes, or holes, are arranged near the tip of the catheter, so as to allow of the passage of liquids to and from its interior. It is better, in metallic as well as in gumelastic instruments, to have two large eyes, not exactly opposite to one another, than to have several rows of minute openings, as was formerly the custom; these small holes being much more apt to become clogged by rust or other causes.

Fig. 125.

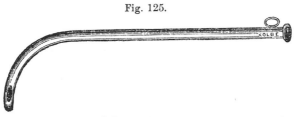

Ordinary male catheter.

On either side of the handle or straight extremity of the silver catheter is fixed a small ring. By the transverse position of these rings, the surgeon knows that the curved extremity of the instrument is passing along the urethra in the median plane; they serve also for the attachment of bands to retain it when it is to be kept in the bladder, as will be mentioned presently. The guide in passing the gum catheter is a ring at the upper end of the iron wire or stilette.

Catheters are made of various sizes. The French scale is numbered from 1 to 30, the English from 1 to 15; the lowest number corresponding to the smallest size. The extremely fine instruments are however very seldom used, and are apt, unless in very skilful hands, to do harm; the largest ones are equally seldom needed. For all ordinary cases, the six or eight medium sizes are sufficient.

A well-rounded tip is a very important advantage in a catheter, being much less apt to injure the mucous membrane lining the canal; but great care is always necessary in using any instrument, especially if resistance is met with.

The use of the catheter is called for when the walls of the bladder lose their tone, so that the urine collects in the viscus, as in old people: when, as in cases of typhoid fever, injuries of the brain, etc., the reflex actions are imperfect: when spasmodic or permanent stricture of the urethra exists: when the neck of the bladder is blocked up by an enlarged prostate, by the pressure of the gravid uterus, or by the lodgment of a small calculus: when rupture of the urethra has taken place: and when for any reason it is desirable to wash out the bladder, or to make applications directly to its mucous surface.

Method of introduction.—The patient may lie on his back, his shoulders slightly raised, his thighs drawn up somewhat, and his knees well apart; the surgeon may stand on either side of him, but can generally operate better if on his left.—Or the patient may sit on the very edge of the bed, his knees wide apart, and his feet on a stool, while the surgeon sits on a chair directly in front of him.—When, from the circumstances of the case or from previous experience, no difficulty is expected in the operation, the patient may simply stand in front of the surgeon, the latter sitting in a chair. It is however unpleasant to both parties if any change has to be made after the operation is begun, and therefore the sitting or lying posture should generally be chosen.

The surgeon now raises the penis lightly between the middle and two last fingers of his left hand, and with the thumb and finger retracts the prepuce if necessary.— Holding the catheter, dipped in oil, lard, cold-cream or any other bland and unirritating lubricant, in his right, he inserts its extremity between the lips of the urethral orifice, and allows it to follow the course of the canal. Often the instrument will catch in the large follicle which is apt to exist on the upper wall of the urethra within the glans; but it is easily disengaged, and by a slight rocking motion carried past this point. The force applied by the surgeon's hand should be most carefully proportioned to the resistance met with. A healthy urethra, especially if the operation has been previously performed, will as it were swallow the catheter. If, as is often the case in old men, the prostate gland is enlarged, the handle of the instrument must be depressed so as to let the tip ride over the elevation and enter the bladder.

The success of the operation is announced to the surgeon by three circumstances. In the first place any resistance that may have been felt ceases, the instrument slipping forward a little of itself, while its handle may be readily depressed. Secondly, the vesical end of the instrument may be moved in any direction by rotating the handle. Thirdly, urine escapes in greater or less quantity; this latter proof is unmistakable.

In very fat subjects, it may be necessary to hold the catheter transversely in first introducing it, to avoid the protuberance of the belly. Or a plan may be resorted to, which was once in great repute, and called the *tour de maître;* the convexity of the curve of the catheter

being directed upwards, and its straight extremity between the patient's thighs, until, as the point progresses
along the canal, the instrument is made to describe a
rotary sweep into the ordinary position.

Should resistance be met with, the surgeon tightens
his hold both on the penis and on the catheter, and pushes
steadily, with very gentle force, against the obstruction.
Sometimes a few moments' perseverance will be rewarded
with success. When this does not occur, a smaller instrument may be tried in the same way. A large instrument, however, sometimes answers better than a small
one, and is certainly safer in inexperienced hands.

To inject the bladder, either with warm water alone
or with medicated washes, we may make use either of an
ordinary catheter, with a syringe fitted to it, the latter
being removed to allow of the escape of the liquid, or of
a double one, bifurcated at its open end so that as the
injection is made through one tube the contents of the
bladder may flow out through the other. This operation, however, is not very frequently called for.

Fig. 126.

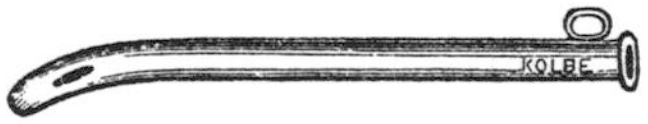

Female catheter.

In the female, a catheter only six or eight inches long,
and very slightly bent near its extremity, is employed.
The only difficulty in its introduction is in finding the
urethral orifice. No exposure of the patient's person is
necessary. The surgeon passes his left hand under the
bedclothes, over the space between the upper part of the
thighs, and then dropping his forefinger backwards into
the vulva, finds the tubercle marking the urethral orifice,

a little below the commissure of the nymphæ. Now, keeping the pulp of this finger on the spot, he carries the catheter, properly lubricated, under the bedclothes with the right hand; it is held tightly between the thumb and the last three fingers, the forefinger being applied to close the orifice. The tip of the instrument is passed along the left forefinger into the urethra; the left hand is now released, and may be used to place a vessel to receive the urine, which flows as soon as the right forefinger is removed from the upper end of the catheter.

In pregnant women, the bladder is drawn up as the uterus becomes developed, so that the orifice of the urethra is sometimes found far up behind the symphysis pubis. The handle of the female catheter would therefore have to be greatly depressed in order to insert its other extremity; and under such circumstances it is often better to use the same instrument as for the male.

After use, a catheter should always be carefully cleansed. It is better, while a case likely to require the trial of several instruments, as for instance one of retention from stricture, is being dealt with, to have a basin of warm water at hand in which to put the catheters as they are laid aside by the surgeon. When all are done with, or whenever the assistant whose duty it is to clean them has an opportunity, they should be taken up one by one, the water poured from the upper end, the freedom of the bore ascertained by blowing through it, and each instrument wiped dry and put in its place.

When it is desirable to retain a catheter in the urethra, it must of course be attached in some way to the body. Silver instruments are best for this purpose, as less likely to be acted upon by the urine; they are also more easily fastened. A gum-elastic catheter of good quality, especially if seasoned by age, may however remain in the urethra for several days without undergoing any change.—The following is the best way to confine an instrument in place in the male: Take a ring of any ma-

Fig. 127.

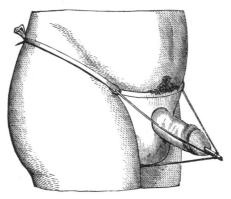

Mode of retaining a catheter in the bladder.

terial, large enough to surround the penis easily even in a state of erection; or if nothing of this kind can be had, make a loop of tape or string. Fasten one part of the catheter to this, by strings or tapes to the rings if the instrument be of silver, by adhesive plaster if it is of gum-elastic. Now attach the ring or loop to the body by adhesive strips, or to a belt round the waist by tapes running directly up in front as well as under the perineum. An arrangement something like this is shown in *Fig.* 127.

The same means, slightly modified, will answer when the catheter is to be retained in the female urethra.

The annexed cut shows the form of catheter employed by Dr. J. Marion Sims, of New York, after operations for vesico-vaginal fistula.

Fig. 128.

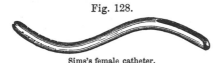

Sims's female catheter.

Bougies are employed for the examination or relief of strictures. They may be made of steel, of soft metallic compounds, of gum-elastic, or of waxed cloth; gutta-percha and whalebone have also been used. Pure tin has been recommended by some authors, as cheaper than silver, and quite as good. When made of steel, these instruments are sometimes provided with a flat roughened handle, or they may be double, the ends being of different sizes; they have as near as may be the curve of the catheter. The soft or flexible metal ones are always double, as are those of waxed cloth; those made of gum-elastic and gutta-percha are usually tipped at the handle with a bit of sealing-wax.

Bougies may have their extremities simply rounded, or conical, or tapering to a fine point, or bulbous or button-pointed. Those of the latter form are most generally made of steel, and are used to ascertain the length of strictures.

The mode of introduction of these instruments does not differ materially from that already described for catheters. Perhaps no operation in surgery demands greater tact, skill or judgment, than this; but these qualities can only be acquired by practice, together with careful study of the pathology of strictures,—a subject with which we are not here concerned.

Bougies are retained in the urethra, when necessary, just as catheters are.

Sounds are used to search for urethral or vesical calculi; they are always made of steel, with flat roughened handles, and in their shapes and sizes do not differ from catheters. Some operators, especially in clinical teaching, employ a flat thin disc of some light wood, fitted by its centre close to the handle of the instrument, to intensify the clicking noise produced when the sound strikes upon a stone.

The *staff* used in lithotomy is made of steel, very much like a sound, but has a groove a little to the right of the median line, along its convexity, terminating a little above the point. Its description, mode of use, etc. belong to the subject of stone in the bladder.

Other instruments, such as the porte-caustique of Lallemand, and those contrived for the incision or dilatation of strictures, are employed; they do not differ in the mode of their introduction from the ordinary catheter, and are more properly described in connection with the morbid states requiring their use.

Catheterization of the Eustachian tube is an operation very rarely called for. M. Guérin* gives the following directions for its performance: "The patient is seated in a chair, his head thrown backward against the chest of an assistant, who holds it firmly between his hands; the surgeon stands in front of him, and taking in his right hand a sound shaped like a female catheter, open at both

---

* Eléments de Chirurgie Opératoire, p. 362.

ends, introduces it by the nostril corresponding to the tube to be entered, passes it from before backwards, the beak of the instrument being turned downwards and outwards, and consequently sliding along the inferior meatus of the nose, its convexity being towards the septum. The sound having passed the bony palate, as is known by the patient making an effort to swallow at the moment, the surgeon raises the point of the instrument slightly, and by moving it still backwards close to the outer wall of the nasal fossa, directs it to the orifice of the Eustachian tube."

A modification of this operation is mentioned by M. Guérin as practised by him, viz., to introduce the forefinger of the surgeon's left hand through the mouth, behind the soft palate, and under the tubercle at the lower edge of the orifice of the tube; this serves as a guide for the end of the instrument. A few introductions of the finger alone, previous to the operation, will enable the patient to bear it without annoyance.

INJECTIONS.—This term needs no explanation, being in popular use.

(1) Injections into the rectum are called also *enemata*, *clysters* or *glysters*, and *lavements*, the latter word being a French one but half naturalized. They may be either simple, or medicated.

Simple enemata are used mainly for the purpose of unloading the large intestine; they consist of water, warm or cold, with or without the addition of a little salt, molasses, soap or starch. Almost always, we prefer warm water, but sometimes, in cases of hæmorrhoids or prolapsus ani, cold or rather cool water may be employed for its sedative and astringent effect; a small quantity is then generally thrown in. The temperature of an enema can hardly be lowered below 45° Fahr. with safety.

Medicated liquids are injected into the rectum for various purposes. A powerful counter-irritant or derivative effect is obtained in cases of congestion or undue excitement of the brain, by the use of a turpentine mixture; one part of Sp. Terebinth. being added to fifteen, ten or five of starch-water or soap-suds. By throwing in from gtt. xl to fʒj of Tr. Opii, with fʒij of starch-water, we may soothe the system at large; this plan is also resorted to in many cases of diarrhœa and dysentery with great benefit. Other anodynes may be used in an analogous way. In some cases of extreme exhaustion, nutritive enemata, composed of beef-essence, strong soups, etc., are employed; the addition to these of a small proportion of pepsine has lately been proposed in imitation of the natural digestive process. Local medication of the large intestine, in cases of dysentery, by means of solutions of nitrate of silver, is often practised.

In all these instances, the mechanical procedure is the same. Syringes of various kinds and sizes are used. The old pewter one has been in a great measure superseded by improved forms, most of which act on the principle of the force-pump. By far the best one yet invented is that known as Davidson's, consisting of two India-rubber tubes attached one to either side of a ball of the same material. Valves are so arranged at the points of attachment that when one end of the apparatus is placed under water, and the bulb alternately squeezed and allowed to expand, the water will be drawn through and forced out at the other end.

Certain points must always be attended to in administering injections into the bowels. The patient will be most conveniently placed in the recumbent position, either on the right or left side, with his uppermost leg and thigh drawn up, just as for the operation for piles or fistula in ano. A tube with a well-rounded bulbous extremity should be employed; it ought to be so large that the mucous membrane will be in no danger of laceration by it.* All the air contained in the instrument should be first expelled, by substituting for it the liquid to be thrown into the bowel. The tip of the left forefinger, carefully oiled, is next to be placed just within the sphincter, to serve as a guide in the introduction of the tube, which should also be duly warmed and oiled. When there is much irritation in the lower bowel, the sphincter is apt to resist, sometimes quite powerfully; firm but gentle pressure must then be used to overcome this resistance. If the syringe is of the old form, the operator must now grasp the body of it firmly with one hand, while with the other he pushes the piston-handle steadily forward, using just as much force as is necessary to move it, and no more. If any variety of the pump be used, the mode of procedure is evident.

Let it never be forgotten that if for any reason we wish to have the injected liquid retained for some length of time, we must throw it in slowly. Thus anodyne enemata should be introduced with the greatest gentleness; the tube should be most carefully inserted, and

---

* When the usual bulk of the fæcal mass as expelled is considered, it will be seen that the sphincter ani is capable of allowing a much larger tube to pass than is commonly employed.

withdrawn as if by stealth. So also when the object is
to soften down a hard fæcal accumulation, the liquid
should be injected slowly, so that it may be retained
until it has permeated the whole mass.

Great care should be observed to avoid giving the
patient pain, or injuring the mucous membrane by any
careless or inadvertent movements of the pipe. When,
as sometimes happens, we wish to apply a solution of
nitrate of silver to the rectum, we may best make use
of a syringe of hard rubber, of any desired capacity.
Or, in default of this, a common glass syringe may answer the purpose. The mechanical procedure is exactly
the same as in other cases; the injection must be accomplished slowly, since we wish the medicated liquid to
remain some little time in contact with the mucous membrane.

(2) Injections into the male *urethra* are used chiefly
in cases of gonorrhœa. The syringe is held by its body,
between the thumb and the three last fingers of the
right hand, the forefinger being kept free to push down
the piston. The tube is inserted in the urethra, as far
as it will go, and held by the thumb and one or two
fingers of the left hand, compressing the glans around it
so as to prevent the escape of any of the liquid when
thrown in. In this manner a system is formed of the
two hands and the charged instrument; the right forefinger is now steadily depressed upon the upper end of
the piston-handle, with a force exactly proportionate
to the resistance met with. When the object in view is
to wash out the bladder, a catheter is first introduced
into that organ, and the stream driven through it by
means of a syringe. A catheter with a double orifice

at the upper end is preferred by some, so that the stream can be passed into the bladder, and escape directly.

(3) Injections into the *vagina* are very seldom administered by the surgeon. The only precaution to be observed is to introduce the instrument far enough to bring the liquid injected into contact with every portion of the cavity.

CHAPTER X.

FOREIGN BODIES.

1. *In the Skin.*—Washerwomen are very apt to get needles stuck in their hands, creeping children are apt to get them in their hands or their knees, and those who go about barefoot get them in their feet. Part of the needle only may enter, the rest either projecting or being broken off. It may pass in entirely, and if it takes up a position lengthwise in an intermuscular space, it may remain a long time without giving any trouble. Sooner or later, however, it will be dislodged, and find its way toward the surface or into some cavity. Splinters of wood in the skin are very common, and although usually very trifling, their extraction may be a matter of difficulty as well as of importance. Other bodies of irregular shape, such as stones, bits of glass, or grains of powder, are apt to become embedded in the skin, especially in railroad accidents, explosions, etc.

Needles and splinters may sometimes be removed by simply pressing on the adjacent skin in such a manner as to make them pierce it outwards. The surgeon should never cut down at hazard, in the hope that he may hit the spot where the needle is, nor should he forget to consider what nerves, vessels, or tendons he may divide in making his incision. He should first distinctly feel the foreign body, and fix it by pressing with the thumb and fingers of the left hand on the skin; he

(232)

should then cut down upon it at some portion of its length, having a pair of suitable forceps at hand with which to grasp it at once. It is surprising how easily the *point* of a needle, beneath the skin, slips away and eludes the knife; and nothing is more awkward for the surgeon, or more painful to the patient, than the necessity of repeated attempts of this kind. Here, as in all other cases, the cuts should be made quite as freely as is needed, but no more; and they should correspond if possible with the natural lines of the skin. Upon the discovery of irregular foreign bodies beneath the skin, which often is only after the occurrence of suppuration, they should be cut down upon and freely extracted.

Grains of powder, if unremoved, cause of course indelible spots. When they are embedded in the skin of the face or hand, they may often be picked out, if the attempt be made early, and they are not in too large numbers; much deformity may in this way be obviated. If the grains are very numerous, another plan may be tried, but it must be done at once; a blister is laid over the affected part, left on from one to four hours, and then followed by a poultice. This method is said to have succeeded in some bad cases.

2. *In the Eye.*—Stone-cutters are very apt to catch minute particles of steel or of stone, struck off as they work, upon the cornea. Great pain and intolerance of light ensue at once, and usually last until the removal of the disturbing cause. This may in most cases be effected by resting the patient's head, thrown far back, against the operator's breast, letting the light strike across the cornea; the little particle being thus seen, the point of a bistoury or a cataract needle may be so

applied, with a steady hand, as to prize it out of its bed. Particles of dust lying on the conjunctiva may generally be seen when the lids are everted, and may be removed either with the blunt end of a probe or by the gentle use of a soft camel's-hair pencil. Should a bit of lime get into the eye, it should of course be removed as early as possible; repeated washings with greatly diluted vinegar will tend to prevent subsequent trouble. A drop or two of castor oil between the lids has a very soothing effect after these accidents. In order to evert the upper lid, the surgeon applies the terminal inch of a probe on the outside of it, just above the upper edge of the palpebral cartilage; then with the thumb and forefinger of the other hand he takes hold of the eyelashes, and drawing the cartilage forwards, gives its edge a sudden sweep upwards, bearing a little downwards at the same time with the probe. The conjunctiva lining the lower lid may be thoroughly inspected by simply drawing down the lid.

3. *In the Ear.*—Children often amuse themselves by stuffing peas, beans, bits of slate pencil, and such small articles, into their own ears or those of their playmates. The surgeon should lose no time in getting anything of the kind away; if the foreign body is soft, like a bean, it is apt to swell with the heat and moisture of the part, and cause dreadful suffering, while if it is hard, the soft tissues lining the ear may become inflamed and swollen. Etherization is almost always necessary in these cases, especially in those of children, and if attempts have been previously made at extraction. Sometimes a stream of tepid water, forcibly driven into the ear, will bring away the foreign body; if this fail, a scoop, a

probe more or less curved, or a fine pair of forceps, may be tried with success. Various forms of forceps have been devised for this purpose. Toynbee's resemble the ordinary dissecting forceps, except in being longer and very narrow, and bent at nearly a right angle just below the middle, so that the operator's hand may not obstruct his view; another form of this instrument has a joint and ring-handles, like a pair of scissors. Dr. Hewson of this city has employed a forceps made on the plan of the ordinary obstetric forceps, in two blades,

Fig. 129.

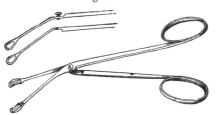

which can be taken apart and introduced separately. Dr. Corse, also of this city, contrived a few years ago an instrument of a simpler shape, the delicate blades being segments of a long narrow cylinder; the anterior one being first introduced, and then the posterior, a small solid "fulcrum" of a cylindrical shape is placed between their outer ends, slit lengthwise to receive two corresponding buttons on the fulcrum. The operator now grasps the instrument, thus put together, and by a gentle but firm to-and-fro motion withdraws it along with the foreign body.* Still another form is the canula

* For a fuller description of this instrument, with a cut, see the *Transactions of the College of Physicians of Philadelphia*, in the *American Journal of the Medical Sciences*, Oct., 1858.

forceps; a pair of blades, opening by a spring, are enclosed in a small canula; they can be pushed out by
means of a slide, and closed upon the foreign body by
pushing the canula forward upon them. This instrument does not work so well as the others, while it is at
the same time more complex, and more apt to get rusty
or otherwise out of order.

Insects are apt to get into the meatus externus; flies
have been known to lay their eggs there, and these to be
developed into maggots. To get rid of any intruders
of this kind, the best plan is to pour a little sweet oil
into the ear, when they will speedily die. Forcible
syringing with soap and water will now dislodge them.

Under this head it may be as well to speak of the
removal of collections of hardened wax from the ears.
Mere syringing will not always effect this; but it will
do so if preceded by the dropping in of some glycerine
or sweet oil, allowing time for this to soften the wax.
Sometimes the operation has to be repeated again and
again before it is completely successful.

4. *In the Nose.*—These cases almost always occur in
children, who insert beans or similar articles into the
nostrils for amusement. When removal with forceps is
difficult or impossible, the surgeon may hold the child's
lips, or have them held, firmly together, while energetic
sneezing is induced by means of snuff or some other
sternutatory. The vapor of liquor ammoniæ, white
hellebore in powder, or the turpeth mineral (yellow
sulphate of mercury) are the articles chiefly used for
this purpose.

5. *In the Trachea.*—By a sudden inspiration, coins,

pins, or any small bodies held in the mouth may be drawn past the rima glottidis. More or less pain and dyspnœa immediately occur, and in the paroxysms of coughing which are apt to ensue the foreign body may be expelled. The common remedy of slapping on the back may aid the expulsive efforts of nature. Another simple plan is to invert the patient more or less completely, putting his feet higher than his head ; this was successful after several trials in the case of the distinguished engineer, Brunel. Tracheotomy is justified and even called for when the foreign body can be made out to be anywhere between the rima glottidis and the lung-substance, and when, other expedients having failed, the dyspnœa and pain are still severe. It had however been ineffectually performed in Mr. Brunel's case, and the coin which he had inhaled was finally expelled by the natural canal. Should the foreign body not escape by the wound made in the operation, very careful search may be made for it with a long and very blunt-ended probe, and a suitable pair of forceps may be used to seize and withdraw it.

6. *In the Pharynx and Œsophagus.*—Pieces of food, swallowed without sufficient chewing, may be arrested in their way to the stomach; this often happens in the paralytic or weak-minded, and hence is a common accident in insane hospitals. During the taking of chloroform or ether, if there is any food in the stomach, it will be rejected; and by lodging in the œsophagus or pharynx may cause death. Or coins or other articles held in the mouth are swallowed, as for instance by the patient laughing suddenly. When respiration is interfered with so as to threaten life, prompt action is of course called for;

the surgeon should first pass his fingers as far down the pharynx as possible, and endeavor to hook the offending mass out, or to cause it to be vomited up. Failing in this, he should pass a probang, tipped with an ivory ball, (the common sponge probang may be made to answer,) or a stomach-tube, or a long rectum-tube, so as to push the mass onward into the stomach. The necessity of subsequent gastrotomy, should the nature of the foreign body be such as to render it probable, would of course be better than the certainty of instant death. If the danger is less imminent, Bond's gullet-forceps, or the whalebone probang with a recurved eye, may be used to entangle the foreign body and draw it up. With a long piece of strong wire, the surgeon may easily make a substitute for this probang as found in the shops. Should it be found impossible to move the foreign body either upwards or downwards, the œsophagus must be opened, according to the usual rules.

Subsequent inflammation should be prevented or allayed by means of mucilages taken by the mouth.

7. *In the Urethra and Bladder.*—Strange as it may seem, there are persons who find satisfaction in inserting sticks, slate-pencils and such bodies into the urethra. Women have often been known to use hair-pins for the purpose. Sometimes the plaything breaks while it is in, or it suddenly slips along the urethra by a sort of suction-power which that tube possesses. If the foreign body reaches the bladder, it excites irritation and inflammation in that viscus, and may become the nucleus of a stone; the salts contained in the muco-purulent secretion poured out becoming encrusted upon it. Gutta-percha bougies are seldom or never employed, on ac-

count of the brittleness they acquire when kept, and their consequent liability to break off while in use.

The female urethra, as is well known, admits of great dilatation; and hence the extraction of foreign bodies from it may be often accomplished with no great difficulty.

If anything becomes lodged near the orifice of the male urethra, attempts may be made to grasp it with fine forceps, or to dilate the tube with some one of the instruments sold for that purpose. The difficulty increases the further back the foreign body is lodged. —A very good plan is to pass the largest possible catheter or bougie down to it, hoping that the expulsive efforts of the bladder upon the accumulated urine may free the canal thus dilated, when the instrument is withdrawn.—Urethral forceps, jointed curettes, etc. have been proposed by Leroy d'Etiolles and others, for catching or grasping the foreign body. Rather, however, than prolong attempts of this kind, the surgeon should push the foreign body back into the membranous portion of the canal, and remove it through an incision made for the purpose; wounds at this point closing better than those anterior to the bulb.—And if this cannot be done, and the bladder is becoming distended, it is better to cut down at once and extract the cause of the trouble, than to risk extravasation of urine.

8. *In the Rectum and Vagina.*—Cases of this kind sometimes require much judgment and mechanical skill. No rules of universal application can be laid down, but the surgeon must remember that his great aim should be to protect the mucous membranes. When glass pessaries or syringes break in the vagina, a common tube specu-

lum may be gently and slowly introduced, the surgeon using a long probe, or a large camel's-hair pencil at the end of a long handle, to wipe the pieces successively brought into view into the instrument. The utmost patience and care are required in such operations, and no forceps or other entangling instrument should ever be introduced unless either guided by the finger or watched by means of the speculum.

It sometimes happens that small bodies, such as fish-bones, pass along the whole alimentary canal without causing any trouble, until they arrive at the anus, when they are arrested by the sphincter, and may find their way into the cellular tissue, an abscess forming around them. Or such a body as a grape-seed may lodge in one of the little pouches which often exist between the columns of the rectum, and cause inflammation and ulceration. Careful examination with the finger will generally reveal the nature of the trouble, and the mode of relief will suggest itself. Should the case have progressed so far that an abscess is manifest externally at the border of the anus, it will be better in opening this abscess to carry the cut through the sphincter at once, so as to prevent the necessity of a subsequent operation for fistula.

CHAPTER XI.

POST-MORTEM EXAMINATIONS.

UNLESS made with accuracy and system, these lose much of their value. Reference ought always if possible to be had to the symptoms presented during life; and notes should be taken at the time the examination is made. In every hospital, a book should be kept for this purpose. The name, age, diagnosis, length of time since death, main characters of the body, as muscular development, emaciation, etc., and degree of rigor mortis, should be noted. Wounds, and all other external marks, should be examined and recorded, especially in cases likely to undergo legal investigation.

The instruments required for the making of a post-mortem are usually kept packed in a case, and are as follows: Three or four scalpels, a heavy cartilage-knife,

Fig. 130.

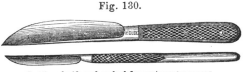

Cartilage-knife and scalpel for post-mortem cases.

a pair or two of dissecting forceps, scissors, a saw, hammer, chisel, rachitome, enterotome, needles, and thread. The scalpels should be of medium size, and it is well that one of them should have a probe point. I use also one curved on the flat, for removing the pelvic viscera.

Some cases are provided with a "brain-knife," thin but
not sharp, about 9 inches long by 1½ wide, rounded at the

Fig. 131.

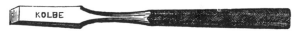

Brain-knife.

end, for slicing the brain. A large electro-plated steel
director is often of service. The saw need not differ
from that ordinarily used in amputations, but is sometimes provided with a shoulder to prevent its cutting too

Fig. 132.

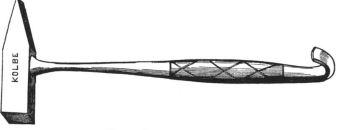

Hammer for post-mortem cases.

deeply in opening the skull; the hammer has an iron
handle curved into a hoop at the end, and a head with

Fig. 133.

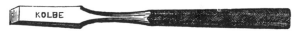

Chisel for post-mortem cases.

one extremity wedge-shaped. The chisel has a short steel
handle. The *rachitome* is a piece of steel shaped as is

seen in *Figs.* 134 and 135, carrying a blunt edge, which
by strokes with a hammer is made to break up the laminæ

Fig. 134.

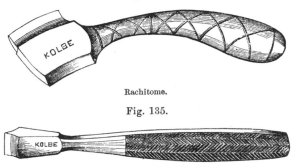

Rachitome.

Fig. 135.

Another form of rachitome.

of the vertebræ so as to expose the spinal cord; it is kept
steady by means of a straight or curved handle attached
to it.   The *enterotome* is merely a large pair of scissors
for laying open the intestinal tube.   One of its blades
is longer than the other, and furnished at the end with a
very blunt hook inclined backwards; this blade is the one
which is put inside the tube, the hook preventing it from

Fig. 136.

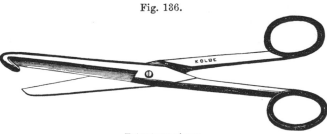

Enterotome scissors.

slipping out as the successive cuts are made.   There is
nothing peculiar about the needles, which are used to

sew up the incisions made, except that they are usually
very large, and roughened in the shank to prevent the
fingers from slipping.

Besides these instruments, there is sometimes supplied
a *costotome*, or pair of cutting pliers with one blunt
point, for dividing the costal cartilages.

The post-mortem case ought always to be kept carefully in order, and the instruments in condition for use.

General directions only can be given here for the
making of autopsies; much must depend on the circumstances of each case, and upon the experience, ingenuity
and skill of the operator. The great object in view is,
of course, to acquire a thorough knowledge of the morbid changes which have been going on during life; but
we must also be careful, especially in private houses, to
avoid any disfigurement of the corpse, as well as all
unnecessary soiling of the dead-clothes, furniture, carpet, etc.

The *brain* should always be examined first, if at all;
since if the other cavities are opened before the cranial,
the atmospheric pressure is taken off, and the blood may
flow away from the cerebral vessels. The hair being
combed back and forward, so as to leave a "part" running from ear to ear across the top of the head, the skin
is divided in the same line, and turned down over the
forehead and occiput. When the hair grows down as
low as usual on the forehead, the scalp should be
loosened not quite as far as its edge. All the soft parts
should then be divided in the line shown in *Fig.* 137,
the skull sawn through all round, and then the calvaria
pried up with the edge of the chisel. Sometimes it will
come away easily, sometimes it adheres very strongly
to the dura mater. The dura mater being now divided

in the same line, the brain is removed by gently passing
one hand under the anterior
cerebral lobes so as to raise
them, while with a knife held
in the other the optic and
other cranial nerves, the
tentorium, and the spinal
cord are successively sev-
ered.   Everything being
clear, the operator lays
down his knife, and holds
one hand to receive the organ, gently turned out into
it with the other.   The organ having been examined,
and as much of it as possible being replaced, the skull
cap is put on, and the divided portions of the temporal
fascia sewn together to keep it steady.   Another plan is
to use bits of stiff wire, inserted into awl-holes made in
the diploë at corresponding points.   But if the saw-cut
has been carefully made according to the directions
above given, these fastenings will be unnecessary.   The
divided edges of the scalp are next sewed together, by
the continuous suture, the thread being carried from
within outwards; and lastly, the hair is combed into its
place again.

Fig. 137.

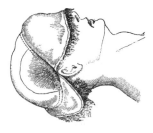

Line of division of the skull in post-
mortem examinations.

The *spinal cord* is best examined by laying the body
on its face, making an incision of sufficient length along
the spinous processes, turning its edges aside, and dividing the vertebral laminæ on either side so as to break
away the arches; a few touches with the knife will then
free all that conceals the dura mater.

To examine the *orbit*, as in cases of suspected disease
within it, the orbital plate of the frontal bone may be

chiseled away, the skull-cap having of course been previously removed. The *eyeball* and its appendages may
be removed in this way, or by separating the eyelids and
emptying the orbit as in an ordinary extirpation.

The *temporal bone* can be taken out for examination,
as in cases of disease of the ear, by dissecting away the
auricle along with the skin, cutting through the zygoma
with bone-forceps, and then sawing down through the
occipital bone close to the suture, and through the
squamous portion in front; a little force will now break
up the bony attachments, and a few touches of the knife
will divide the soft parts.

The contents of the mouth may be easily removed for
examination by means of a single incision from the
hyoid bone down the median line.

The *thoracic and abdominal viscera* are best examined
by taking them all out together, any abnormities of attachment or relation to the parietes being first looked
for. An incision is made from the interclavicular notch
to the pubes, along the median line, avoiding the umbilicus. The sternum and costal cartilages are next laid
bare by rapid dissection; the knife is carried through
the sterno-clavicular articulation on either side, down
through the cartilages at each side close to their junction
with the ribs, and through the soft parts attached to the
front lower edge of the thorax. The "breast-plate" is
now lifted and turned back over the face, the areolar
tissue being dissected away close to the bone, and
by cutting through the abdominal muscles and fasciæ
transversely, opposite the umbilicus, the skin is freed so
that the two great cavities of the trunk are completely
open for study.

Before proceeding further, the state of the pleural

cavities as to the amount and character of the contained liquid, the adhesions existing, etc. should be noted; and the operator should insinuate his hand around the lungs so as to free them if they are attached anywhere. Next, drawing down the trachea and œsophagus at the root of the neck, he divides them with the large vessels, and carries the dissection down along the spinal column, pulling the viscera forwards and separating them now with the knife and now with the fingers. Dividing the diaphragm all around at its costal attachment, he proceeds to draw forward and free the liver, duodenum, kidneys and mesentery; a ligature is placed upon the rectum, and the gut cut across below it, when the whole mass of the viscera may be removed.

When tumors, such as large aneurisms, cysts, etc. are present, it is better to study them as much as possible *in situ*. For cases where the pelvic viscera are diseased to any extent, I use a knife curved on the flat, to be carried right round the concavity of the bones, and separate everything; this can hardly be done neatly with a straight scalpel.

To examine any tubular parts,—the bronchi, vessels, or intestinal canal,—the enterotome, a pair of probe-pointed scissors, or a probe-pointed knife, may be used according to circumstances. The solid viscera are studied by making sections into them, and by tearing.

For some of the hollow viscera special modes of opening must be adopted.—The *heart's* cavities are exposed as follows: a cut is carried through the anterior wall of the right auricle from the mouth of one vena cava to that of the other, and another cut from this one into the auricular appendage. The finger is now passed into the right ventricle, and the anterior wall of the latter cut

through parallel with and near to the interventricular
septum; another cut is made at an acute angle with this,
and a triangular flap of the wall can be turned up so as
to lay the cavity open.   The finger is now turned upwards and passed into the pulmonary artery, and the
knife guided along it so as to lay this vessel also open,
avoiding the flaps of the semilunar valve.   In an analogous way the left side of the organ may be opened.—
The *stomach* should be laid open by a cut along its
lesser curvature; the *jejunum* and *ileum* by carrying the
enterotome along the line of attachment of the mesentery.—The wall of the *bladder* should always be divided
above, from before backwards.

All that is not to be reserved being returned into the
body, a quantity of bran, of cotton, or of absorbent
paper is also inserted, to take up any liquids which would
otherwise either flow out or putrefy.   The breast-plate is
replaced, and all the cuts that have been made in the
skin are sewed up by means of the continuous or glover's
suture.

Cuts and scratches are very apt to be sustained by
the operator during the making of an autopsy; they seldom amount to anything, but it is safer that the hands
should be at once washed, and the wound well sucked.
More commonly, an old cut or scratch is the channel
of absorption of some noxious material into the system, under circumstances well known, but by no means
understood; the state of health has undoubtedly much
to do with the susceptibility to the poison.

CHAPTER XII.

DISINFECTANTS.

BESIDES the ordinary and well-known contagious or infectious diseases, there are conditions of the system, brought on probably by some atmospheric change, in which it is prepared to receive with special readiness, and to give out again, certain morbific influences. Especially in large and crowded hospitals, and during seasons when the temperature of the air is extremely hot, cold or variable, do we notice this. Dysentery and erysipelas are perhaps the diseases most apt to take on this propagative character.

Again, we sometimes see a tendency prevailing in a hospital, or in a single ward, to the occurrence of phagedæna; every sore already existing becoming gangrenous, and new ones of like character breaking out. This may occur in persons who are isolated, but is far more apt to be met with where a number of patients are collected together. We cannot but attribute it to atmospheric influence, whether we suppose organic particles or *fomites* floating in the air, or adopt a more purely chemical theory, such as that of catalysis.

To combat the conditions now mentioned, we use what are called disinfectants or antiseptics. One class of these, of which chlorine may be taken as the type, acts by chemically decomposing the noxious substance. Another, of which carbon is the main element, would

22 (249)

seem merely to arrest and detain it. Still another class is made up of various articles which stimulate or otherwise influence the tissues to a healthier action. As, however, this classification cannot in practice be maintained with absolute accuracy, we shall merely pass in review the different substances coming under the general denomination of disinfectants or antiseptics.

Chlorine is the best known, and perhaps the most efficient of the disinfectants properly so called. It is readily given off by many of its compounds, and thus becomes diffused in the form of vapor, so as to attack and neutralize any noxious effluvia which may be floating in the air. Chloride of lime may be placed in shallow dishes or trays here and there in the ward or room to be purified; it undergoes change, carbonic acid being taken up from the atmosphere, and chlorine gas slowly given off. In like manner the solution of chlorinated soda (Liq. Sodæ Chlorinatæ of the U. S. Pharmacopœia, known also as "Labarraque's solution") may be sprinkled about. Either of these agents should be used in such a quantity as to cause a decided odor of chlorine. Dysenteric discharges, slop-basins and jars used to contain foul and dirty dressings in a surgical ward, may be freed from all noxious or disagreeable smell by the same means.

On the standard supply table for the army, last issued, will be found " Chlorinium (the materials for preparing.)" For.the following account of these materials I am indebted to the kindness of Dr. R. S. Satterlee, U. S. A., through whom I obtained them from Dr. E. R. Squibb, of Brooklyn.

"(*a*) The *manganese mixture.*—Take of binoxide of

manganese, containing 72 per cent., 1875 parts; common salt, well dried, 1800 parts; and having ground them together into a fine powder, put this up in papers containing about 195 grains each, placing 130 of these papers in a stout pasteboard box labeled with plain directions for use.

"(Should the binoxide of manganese be either richer or poorer than 72 per cent., the quantity must be adjusted accordingly.)

"(b) The *sulphuric acid mixture.*—Take of sulphuric acid, sp. gr. 1·845, 45 parts; water, 21 parts; mix them carefully, allow the mixture to become cold, and put it up in very strong bottles, with accurately ground stoppers, 65 fluidounces in each bottle.

" One of the above powders placed in a saucer or plate, and thoroughly mixed with half a fluidounce of the sulphuric acid mixture, is to be placed under every alternate bed at night, and allowed to remain there one week. Upon the night following the beds omitted the first night are to be supplied in the same way and for the same length of time, and the whole process repeated or continued according to circumstances. Should the wards be badly ventilated, or contain many sloughing wounds, or be subject to epidemic disease, or to low forms of fever, the process should be continuous. Otherwise once or twice a month may be sufficient. When thorough ventilation and cleanliness can be attained, the process is unnecessary for occupied wards.

" In disinfecting unoccupied wards, water-closets, latrines, etc., they should be first cleansed, then closed up as perfectly as possible, and two powders used for each 600 cubic feet of space.

" Each powder, when used as above directed, yields

spontaneously about 57 inches of chlorine. This quantity, thus liberated gradually in a space containing 20,000 times its volume of air, is borne without inconvenience by most persons, and is not injurious even to those laboring under pulmonary disease. As very much depends on the circulation of air, and the ventilation of apartments where it is used, no absolute rules of application can be laid down, except that it should never be used in such quantities as to produce discomfort or bronchial irritation to patients. There are some persons who cannot bear chlorine at all without annoyance, and such should of course be removed from any apartment where it is to be used."

"Burnett's disinfecting fluid," a solution of chloride of zinc in water, 200 grains to the fluidounce, has been very highly recommended as a disinfectant, but is more used in this country, somewhat diluted, for injecting subjects for the dissecting-room.

Chloride of zinc is a well-known caustic, and when dissolved in water, about grs. v to f℥j, an excellent astringent for ulcers which require gentle stimulation. Perhaps the chlorine has some slight corrective effect upon the fetor apt to be observed in the discharge from such ulcers.

It should be mentioned that Labarraque's solution, largely diluted with water, say one part to sixteen or more, forms an admirable dressing for foul wounds or sores. Often after injuries of bone there will be a very copious and offensive discharge of matter, which may even render the air of the room unbearable; and at the same time there is a tendency to exuberant and flabby granulation in the soft parts. The mixture above mentioned, made stronger or weaker according to circumstances, answers an excellent purpose in such cases.

Iodine in the form of vapor is said to have been used as a disinfectant in the Middlesex Hospital, London. About ℈ij of pure iodine are placed in a small box or other convenient receptacle, and hung over the patient's bed.* No trial of this plan has to my knowledge been made in this country as yet.

Carbon is used as a disinfectant under various forms. As smoke, its power in preventing the decomposition of meat is familiar to every one, and it is commonly employed to purify vessels, houses, etc. in which infectious diseases have prevailed. To destroy odors, such as those from fæcal discharges, etc., it is an excellent plan to burn sugar or coffee in the room.

A poultice, made of the finely powdered charcoal of bone, (which is better than that obtained from wood,) will correct entirely the fetor of foul ulcers, gangrenous sores, etc. Creosote, added in small quantity to lotions or to poultices, has much the same power, but it has itself an odor which to some persons is very unpleasant. The oakum dressing, already spoken of,† has a decidedly antiseptic property, due no doubt to the tar it contains; it forms therefore an excellent application for foul sores, while it is slightly astringent and stimulating. In one case under my care, in which an abdominal abscess

---

* The Ambulance Surgeon, or Practical Observations on Gunshot Wounds. By P. L. Appia, M.D., etc. Edinburgh edition, p. 202.

† Chapter I, p. 29.

poured forth an immense quantity of fetid pus, with a strong fæcal odor, the air of the patient's room was intolerable until I began to employ oakum soaked in hot water as a dressing; this corrected the smell entirely.

Nearly allied to creosote in chemical characters is a substance called carbolic acid, lately introduced as a disinfectant. As furnished for army use, it is in combination with several other articles, in the form of a powder. This powder, like chloride of lime, is placed in shallow trays in the room or ward to be purified. Extended trials of it have not yet been made.

Some other substances have been proposed as disinfectants. The sulphite of soda, the double sulphite of soda and iron, the hypochlorite of soda or lime, have had their respective advocates. These may any of them be used in the absence of better proved articles, and may with great propriety be tested in any cases where circumstances do not render the experiment hazardous.

Heat has been resorted to for the purification of clothes, sheets, etc., but is by no means a certain resource. Dry heat is applied by bringing the infected articles to a high temperature in an oven; moist heat, merely by boiling them in water or an alkaline solution. The former is the more effectual plan, but requires careful management.

Ledoyen's disinfecting fluid is a solution of nitrate of lead. It owes its efficiency to its power of decomposing sulphuretted hydrogen, and therefore can have but a limited application.

Nitrous acid fumes, obtained by heating the nitrate of lead, have been recommended for the purification of infected apartments.

Camphor is popularly supposed to possess disinfectant powers, but there is no reason for such an idea. Nor is there any proof that *whitewash*, which has a like reputation, is anything more than a means of cleanliness, and thus an indirect remedy for one of the circumstances favoring the propagation of disease.

Of the articles employed for changing the character of the surface in foul or sloughing sores, we have quite a variety.—*Nitrate of silver*, in the solid stick or in solution, is very useful when there is merely a tendency to gangrene; its action is superficial only.—*Nitric acid*, applied in its full strength, causes a much deeper slough to come away, and the surface left will often be found healthy. Very much diluted, (50 minims to Oj of water,) it may be used as a wash, once or twice daily, with the happiest effect.—The *permanganate of potash*, in solution, forms an excellent lotion for unhealthy and foul smelling wounds or sores.—The disinfecting powder invented by MM. Corne and Demeaux, consisting of 100 parts sulphate of lime and 3 of coal-tar, although not without a certain degree of efficiency, has an unpleasant smell, and has fallen into disuse.—*Lime-water* forms a very good application where an acrid ichorous discharge irritates the surface around an abscess or ulcer. It may be used as a wash, poured over the part, or it may be kept applied by means of soft rags saturated in it, just as any other water-dressing.

It should never be forgotten that these local means

will hardly be of any avail unless constitutional remedies are also employed. There is almost invariably some vice of system manifesting itself in these cases, which must be corrected before any permanent advantage is gained. Quinine, iron in some form, the mineral acids, as well as a generous diet, with malt liquors, are indicated, and would quite probably effect a change in many cases if combined with only the simplest local treatment.

CHAPTER XIII.

ON SOME MINOR OPERATIONS.

UNDER the above heading it has seemed to me proper to place certain surgical procedures which, in their mere performance, are, as a general rule, simple and free from danger. It should be borne in mind, however, that even these may in some cases present difficulties, and be followed by grave consequences; so that due caution should be observed in resorting to them.

I. THE OPENING OF ABSCESSES.—Unless under special circumstances, as for example when formed beneath a dense fascia, the existence of pus is known by the physical sign of *fluctuation;* a wave being transmitted from one finger or one hand to the other, when pressure is alternately made at two opposite points. Care should always be taken not to choose two points in the width of a muscular belly, as otherwise we may be completely deceived, the mass of the muscle yielding transversely exactly as a collection of liquid would.

The presence of pus being determined, the duty of the surgeon almost invariably is to let it out; the exceptions need not be noticed here. The method usually chosen is by incision.

When an abscess is superficial, of moderate size, and especially when it has any specific character, the rule is to lay it open freely. A very large or deep-seated one, on the other hand, should be so opened as to allow as little air as possible to enter its cavity; and the same is true of mammary abscesses, or such as are in places where scars would be inconvenient. In the first case, the surgeon takes a curved sharp-pointed bistoury in his right hand, and with his left steadies the affected part. Now, holding the bistoury with its back downward, he plunges the point through the wall of the abscess, depresses the handle so as to carry the point on as far as he deems proper, thrusts it up and out through the skin by further depressing the handle, and completes the cut by raising the instrument. Hardly an instant is occupied in this act. The hand should be wholly free, so that if the patient starts suddenly the knife may be as quickly moved, and all danger of accident avoided.

In the second case, a straight sharp-pointed bistoury is thrust in perpendicularly to the skin, and rotated a little on its long axis, when the pus will flow up alongside of it; if now the abscess is very deep seated, the muscular and other tissues may be divided by moving the point of the knife to and fro to the desired extent, avoiding, of course, any important vessels and nerves.

Another method is by pinching up a fold of the skin, and carrying a straight sharp-pointed bistoury nearly through its base; then by raising the handle of the instrument its point may be brought into position to be pushed on into the cavity of the abscess. On withdrawing it, a track or sinus will be left for the discharge of matter. Still another method is to pass a seton through as much of the cavity as may be deemed convenient or desirable; the matter will escape beside this as well as by absorption into its substance. Finally, the method of drainage proposed by Chassaignac commends itself for some cases. This is to employ a small India-rubber tube, perforated here and there with holes, either passed through the abscess like a seton, or one end only caused to enter the cavity; the idea being that the pus will flow into the holes and be continually drained away.

Caustics, as a means of opening abscesses, have been almost wholly abandoned at the present day. Some surgeons still employ them for venereal buboes; and some patients would rather undergo any torture than submit to the use of the knife. The surrounding surface being duly protected by means of cerate or adhesive plaster, the caustic is placed upon the skin to be destroyed, and left there until its work is accomplished. Formulæ of the various caustics, Vienna paste, Canquoin's, Filhos's, Manec's, Frére Côme's, Justamond's, the acid nitrate of mercury, etc., may be found in other works, and would be out of place here.

II. The Laying open of Sinuses.—A sinus is a track lined with a more or less definite false membrane, without any disposition to close; it may have either one or two openings, and may have branches leading off from it. Fistula in ano is simply a sinus, sometimes opening both on the skin and into the bowel, sometimes into the bowel only, (blind internal fistula,) sometimes on the skin only, (blind external fistula.)

When on the surface of the body, sinuses are laid open by a very simple process. A director, curved if necessary, is passed along the track, and upon it is introduced a bistoury, so as to divide the bridge of skin. In fistula in ano, we pass the director, curved to the requisite degree, through the canal, bringing it out at the anus; a curved bistoury is then carried along the groove and made to cut its way out. Sometimes, when the sinus is short and wide, the director may be dispensed with, a probe-pointed bistoury being used. If the inner orifice is very high up, we pass a forefinger into the gut, guide the knife through the fistula with a director until its point is engaged against the forefinger, and then bring the finger and knife down together.

III. LIGATURES.—Ligatures are used for the strangulation of abnormal tissues, causing them to slough away by depriving them of their vascular supply. Annealed iron or silver wire, saddler's silk, or any thread of sufficient tenacity, may be employed for the purpose.

When wire is used, it is applied by means of a double canula, consisting of two slender tubes forming one

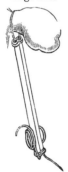

Fig. 138.

Wire applied to the base of a pile by means of a double canula.

stem; a small ring or button is provided at the outside of each tube near its end, and one end of the wire is made fast to one of them. The wire being now passed through the corresponding tube, and back again through the other, a loop is left which may be slipped over the part to be destroyed. The surgeon now draws upon the free end of the wire so as to tighten the loop as strongly as possible, and then fastens it upon the adjacent button; the canula is thus left hanging until the constricted part falls away. This plan is often employed for the cure of hæmorrhoids. Another mode is to fasten both ends of the wire, and then to tighten the loop by means of a screw; the instrument for this purpose is well known as "Græfe's *serre-nœud*." For uterine polypi, a similar plan is followed, but the upper portions of the canula are separate from each other and from the lower part of the instrument, to facilitate the adjustment of the ligature, which is usually composed of fine twine or sea-grass. The instrument thus modified is known as "Gooch's canula."

Various modes of applying thread ligatures have been contrived. The most common application of this form is in the case of hæmorrhoids, or of the nævi, mother-marks or erectile tumors which appear ɔ children at the third or fourth month after birth.

The tying of piles, when small, is easily accomplished by passing a needle armed with a double ligature through the base of the tumor, cutting the thread off at the eye of the needle, and tying the corresponding ends together. A special contrivance known as "Bushe's needle," for carrying the ligature from within the anus outwards, will be found described in works on general surgery. Larger piles or nævi may be strangulated in divided portions by carrying a long thread back and forward so as to make a succession of loops, (*Fig.* 139.) Or when the growth is too broad for this, the needle and double ligature may be carried through in one direction, and the thread cut at the eye of the needle; then one end of the thread may be taken up and carried crosswise, to be again cut

Fig. 139.

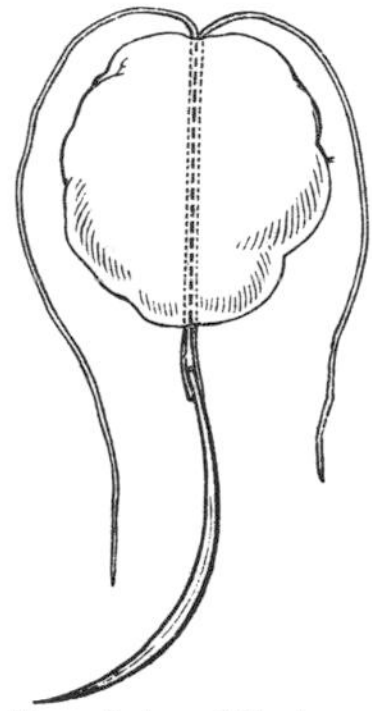

Transfixion of the base of a pile, in order to its ligation.

at the eye of the needle.   Two of the three pair of ends
being now firmly knotted together, the third may be

Fig. 140.   Fig. 141.

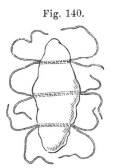

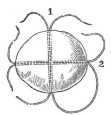

Diagram of tumor with its
base transfixed by a number
of threads.

Diagram of tumor with its
base transfixed by two threads,
at right angles to one another.

strongly drawn and tied, and the whole mass will be
constricted.

Nævi, when small, may be strangulated by passing
two fine hare-lip pins under them at right angles to one
another, each needle entering the sound skin about
one-eighth of an inch from the edge of the tumor, and
emerging at a like distance from it on the other side; a
strong ligature is now cast around under the free ends
of the needles, and tied as firmly as possible.   The
tumor becomes at first intensely red, then dark purple
and cold, and in a few days will drop off, leaving an
ulcerated surface which heals readily.   If the tumor is
of larger size, additional needles may be passed, or one
portion of it may be ligated at a time.

As a substitute for ligation by the thread or wire, as
well as for removal by the knife in many cases, M. Chas-

saignac of Paris several years ago proposed what he
calls *écrasement lineaire*. His *écraseur* is simply a
canula, having a chain loop at one end, and at the other
an arrangement for tightening it gradually but irre-

Fig. 142.

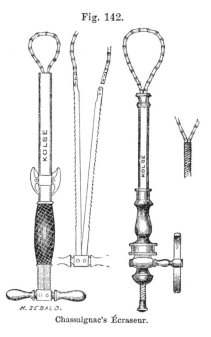

Chassaignac's Écraseur.

sistibly, (*Fig.* 142.) The modus operandi of this instrument will be at once perceived; its special applications,
which are less numerous than was at first supposed, may
be more appropriately defined in other works.

It should not be forgotten that the skin is extremely
sensitive to the pressure of a ligature, and must always
be divided with a knife in the line over which the thread
or twine will pass.

M. Maisonneuve, of Paris, not long since published a memoir on what he calls the "*ligature extemporanée.*" This is simply the use of a very strong thread or wire in the same way as the chain of the écraseur. A screw like that of Græfe's *serre-nœud* is employed to tighten the loop, and the tightening process is carried on until the tissues are cut through. Three sizes of the instrument are described by M. Maisonneuve, to be used according to the degree of force necessary to the desired end.

The *subcutaneous* ligature is sometimes employed for small nævi situated entirely beneath the skin. It is applied by passing a strongly-curved needle, armed with a ligature, through the skin near one edge of the growth, carrying it half way round the latter, and bringing it out. Entering it again at its point of emergence, it is passed around the other half of the tumor, and brought out at its first point of entrance. The growth is now surrounded by a loop, the end of which may be readily drawn tight and tied.

The same principle may be applied to nævi of larger circumference, by making the points of exit and re-entrance of the needle more numerous and at shorter intervals.

IV.—OPERATION FOR HARE-LIP.—Children are sometimes born with the upper lip more or less deficient in the middle, so that their sucking is interfered with, as well as subsequently their articulation. The same state of things may be caused by accident at any period of life. Cases of this kind vary much in their severity; when simple, their treatment comes properly within the limits of minor surgery.

The lip being well freed from the gum, the edges of the cleft must be pared, so as to make two raw surfaces, the end of a thin slip of wood being placed within the lip, and the cut made upon this with a bistoury or scalpel; the twisted or hare-lip suture is then used to keep them together, supported by adhesive strips.

In making the incisions, we should follow two curved lines, their concavities look-ing towards one another, as in the cut; in this way the slight central protru-sion natural to the lip is imitated. Some surgeons prefer curved scissors to the knife for paring the edges, and Mr. Cooper Forster of

Fig. 143.

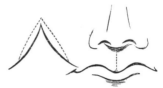

Elliptical incision in the operation for hare-lip.

London recommends the continued instead of the twisted suture.

V. VACCINATION.—The history and objects of this operation are too well known to need mention here. In some countries its performance upon children is enjoined by law; and among civilized nations it is almost universal, although there are many intelligent men in the medical profession who doubt its efficacy as a preventive against small-pox.

Vaccination may be done upon persons of any age; but in my own experience it has seldom been successful in children less than four months old. It consists in the introduction beneath the cuticle, and thus into the cir-culation, of matter from a sore of the same kind as that we wish to produce. The point chosen is generally at the upper part of the arm, the higher the better in female children; that arm being preferred which is habitually kept away from the nurse or mother in carrying.

Should a child be vaccinated which presents any unhealthy phenomena, any eruption, strumous or syphilitic taint, or any general weakness of system, the idea of vaccinating any other child with the matter taken from it should be rejected, simply on prudential grounds. One vaccine scab may propagate itself indefinitely by successive transmissions through healthy children.

Some practitioners employ lymph taken from the vaccine sore when at its height, between the sixth and eighth days; others use the dried scab mixed with a little water. When the lymph is preferred, it is obtained by puncturing the vesicle, and receiving the matter upon a small glass plate; another glass plate is laid upon it, and the edges of the two luted together with wax: to use it, the plates are separated, and a little saliva or water is added to the virus to moisten it. A better plan is to have a small cavity in one of the plates, in which the virus may be lodged; there is then no danger of the two plates adhering too strongly together when it is desirable to separate them. Some practitioners use fine glass tubes, sealed up when charged with the matter from a fresh vaccine sore.—The scab, taken as it drops off when completely mature, is enclosed in wax, collodion, tin foil, or any other convenient envelope, to exclude the air. A little of it is rubbed up with water to the consistence of thin paste, when it is to be used.

The former of these methods is perhaps the better in military practice, or in public institutions, where large numbers are to be operated on at one time; but for private patients the use of the scab will be found more convenient.

Different methods of performing this little operation have been devised. That which I recommend is as follows: The child's sleeve being well secured up on the shoulder, the surgeon scrapes away the cuticle with the edge of a dull thumb-lancet, until red points of vascularity begin to appear. Having thus provided an absorbent surface about ⅜ of an inch in diameter each way, he places upon it a drop of the moistened lymph or scab; this drop is then allowed to dry by exposure to the air.—Another plan is to take a thin sharp-pointed lancet, and insert its tip beneath the cuticle at two or three different points; a small particle of the lymph or scab is then pushed into each of the little pockets so formed, and left to be absorbed.—Another plan is to make a cut through the cuticle just down to the true skin, and in this to lay a thread soaked in the liquefied lymph or scab.—Special instruments have been also invented for passing under the cuticle the pointed end of a fine tube, along which the vaccine matter is pushed by means of a sort of piston.

Whichever of the plans now described is adopted, it is just as well to apply the virus at several points, so as fairly to test the susceptibility of the patient. When the operation succeeds, the part seems for a few days to return to perfect quiescence. "The local signs indicating that the vaccination has taken effect are first apparent on the third or fourth day after the operation, at which period there is a slight degree of elevation and hardness of the skin (papular stage) at the seat of the puncture, and a trifling blush of redness immediately surrounding it. On the fifth and sixth day, a small quantity of liquor sanguinis is effused beneath the epidermis, and a vesicle is formed, which is whitish or pearly in appearance, of a roundish or oval figure, and umbilicated at its centre. The vesicle goes on increasing in size until the eighth or ninth day, at which period it has become fully distended, and has attained its perfect development. On the ninth day it loses the umbilicated form, it becomes flattened on the surface, and sometimes more convex than at the circumference, and is composed of numerous small cells, which are filled with a limpid and transparent lymph.

"On the eighth day, (sometimes the ninth,) the perfect vesicle is surrounded by an inflamed areola, of a vivid red color, (*the pearl upon the rose*,) which gradually increases in extent, from a few lines to more than two inches in diameter. The skin included in this areola is inflamed and tumefied, and is frequently the seat of eruption of a crop of small transparent vesicles. On the tenth day, the redness and heat have increased; there is considerable itching in the part, the movements of the arm are somewhat painful, and the axillary glands are liable to become tender and swollen. It occasionally happens that at this period an erythematous blush spreads from the arm over the surface of the body, in irregular patches.

"On the eleventh day the areola begins to diminish, the fluid contained within the vesicle has become purulent, and desiccation commences at its centre, and proceeds gradually towards the circumference. During the succeeding days the areola disappears more and more, the tumefaction subsides, and the vesicle desiccates into a dark-brownish crust of an irregular form. The crust, by a continuance of desiccation, diminishes in size, and assumes a blackish hue. It is detached at the end of seventeen days after vaccination, and leaves upon the skin a depressed cicatrix, at the bottom of which are seen numerous small pits, (foveolæ,) which correspond with the separate cells of which the vesicle was composed. The cicatrix is permanent, enduring for the remainder of life."*

It sometimes happens that the areola is intensely inflamed and painful; this excessive action is best allayed by sponging gently with cold lead-water, taking care that the vesicle and its forming scab are untouched.

Revaccination is performed in the same manner. It very often fails, but succeeds in a sufficient proportion of cases to establish its importance.

VI. The Introduction of the Seton.—A seton is simply a thread or threads, or a strip of some fabric, passed through a portion of skin, and its ends brought together and tied; wire has been used in the same way. Sometimes this is done merely to excite a local irritation for the relief of trouble existing elsewhere, as at the back of the neck for cerebral congestion; sometimes it is to drain off liquids, as when the seton is made to traverse the cavity of an abscess or of a hydrocele. Sinuses are occasionally treated by drawing a seton through them.

When a wire or a single thread is used, any common suture needle, if long enough, answers to introduce it with; for a number of threads, or a strip of lint or other material, the large and broad "seton-needle" is very convenient.

---

* Wilson on Skin Diseases, Am. ed., p. 460.

But the operation may be quite as readily performed with a straight bistoury and eyed probe, in the following way:—Pinch up with one thumb and forefinger a fold of skin of suitable size, and pass the bistoury transversely through its base ; now carry the probe through along the flat of the bistoury, and withdraw the latter; pass one end of the seton through the eye of the probe, and draw it through just as you would with a needle.

Setons may be rendered more irritating by smearing them with stimulating ointments, or by soaking them in suitable liquids.

VII. The Formation of Issues. — An issue is a small deep ulcer made and kept up by the surgeon. The skin is broken either by means of chloride of zinc, Vienna paste, or some other caustic, or by an incision made obliquely so as to form a small pocket, and this solution of continuity is kept open by the insertion and retention in it of a small foreign body, called an "issue-pea," a piece of wood about as large as a pea being most commonly used.

VIII. The Application of the Moxa. — This is simply a form of the actual cautery, consisting in the burning of some substance in contact with the skin. Nothing is better for the purpose than a little roll of lint steeped in a saturated solution of nitre; the diameter of the cylinder being about half an inch, and its length a little less.

For use, such a cylinder is held in a pair of dressing forceps, one end of it lighted, and the other end applied to the desired spot on the skin; the operator may hasten the combustion by blowing either with the breath or with a blow-pipe. As the heat approaches the surface, there is a gradually increasing sense of warmth, which becomes at length extremely painful; and the skin assumes at that point an opaque whitish-yellow color. In a few days a small slough separates, and leaves a deep ulcer, which constitutes an effective means of counter-irritation, especially if dressed with stimulating ointments or washes.

In cases of spinal disease of limited extent, the moxa is a most valuable remedy, and has fallen too much into disuse. It is an excellent substitute for the actual cautery.

IX. PHYMOSIS AND PARAPHYMOSIS.—*Phymosis* is said to exist when the prepuce cannot be drawn back over the glans penis. It may be due either to congenital formation, to simple inflammatory swelling, or to changes induced by venereal disease. An operation is called for, in congenital cases, to prevent any hindrance to the development of the glans, and to obviate the uncleanliness necessarily resulting from such a condition; in venereal cases, to enable us to deal effectively with any diseased spots concealed within the prepuce. Cases of mere inflammation only need to be operated upon when there is trouble during erection of the penis; otherwise we simply treat the cause.

The operation to be performed in congenital cases, where the glans is comparatively very small, is simply to draw the prepuce forward, to catch it between the blades of a pair of slender forceps, and then with a bistoury to slice away all that projects, (*Fig.* 144.) The mucous

Fig. 144.

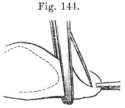

Operation for phymosis.

membrane still remains to be divided, which is done by slitting it up in the median line above with a pair of fine probe-pointed scissors; the scissors are then used again to cut away the angular flap of mucous membrane on either side, and many surgeons fasten the corresponding edges of the skin and mucous membrane together by a few points of suture. The suture is not in my opinion necessary.

In venereal cases, where there are probably ulcers beneath the swollen prepuce, a simple slit along the median line by means of a pair of scissors, one blade being introduced under the membrane, will suffice; two triangular flaps can then be turned off on either side, and the whole diseased surface reached. Healing takes place with very little deformity.

In neither of these operations does any hæmorrhage occur which cannot be readily restrained by pinching the cut edge of the prepuce, or by the application of ice-water.

Paraphymosis is the opposite condition to that just described; the prepuce is retracted and cannot be brought forward. Swelling of the glans takes place, and will, if relief be not given, terminate in gangrene.

When cold water, applied for an hour or two, fails to reduce the swelling, the surgeon must grasp the penis, just back of the glans, between the forefinger and middle finger of each hand, and then, pressing with both thumbs upon the swollen glans, endeavor to lessen its size and push it back within the prepuce.

Failing in this, he must insinuate the probe point of a fine pair of scissors under the tense prepuce, and cut it directly across. It will immediately gape widely, and the reduction of the glans can be readily accomplished.

X. VARICOCELE.—By this term is meant an enlargement of the spermatic veins; although some writers restrict the term to cases where the veins of the scrotum are affected, applying the word *cirsocele* to those in which the disorder is limited to the spermatic cord. The diagnosis is easy.

Palliative measures, such as the use of cooling and astringent lotions, and the fitting of a suspensory bandage, are sometimes resorted to in civil life; but in military practice, and in fact wherever this affection is the only abnormal condition present, an operation may be safely and properly performed.

I shall mention only one, which is so simple and certain as to answer every purpose.

A slender needle about three inches long, having near the point an eye and a slight curve, is threaded with annealed iron wire; a small plate of sheet-lead, about an inch or an inch and a quarter in length, and about half an inch wide, perforated near each end with a round hole, is also provided. The needle may either be set in a handle, or grasped with forceps. The operator isolates the bundle of spermatic veins, and passes the needle *behind* it; he then withdraws the needle, leaving a loop of wire at one side, and two ends at the other. Now, threading the needle again with wire, he passes it in the contrary direction, through the same openings, but *in front* of the veins, and withdraws the needle, leaving the loop as before. Each pair of ends is now passed through the loop of the other, drawn upon, and passed through the holes in the lead-plate, over which they are all twisted together.

XI. Hydrocele.—Hydrocele is an accumulation of serum in the tunica vaginalis testis. This sac surrounds the gland except at its posterior and upper edge, and admits of distension to an enormous degree, so that the mere weight of the swelling may be a source of extreme discomfort.

The diagnosis in these cases is generally made without difficulty. Hernia, hæmatocele, and chronic inflammation or malignant disease of the testis, are the affections most likely to be confounded with hydrocele. But if the tumor is painless, soft, fluctuating, and pyriform, if it is known to have appeared first at the lower part of the scrotum, and if in a darkened room it transmits the light of a candle, a mistake can scarcely be made.

To apply the candle-test, let the room be well darkened; let the patient stand up, and the operator sit on one side and somewhat in front of him. An assistant placed on the other side now brings the flame of a candle as close as possible to the scrotum, while the surgeon applies his open hands by their radial edges so as to shut off any light from his eyes except what passes through the part to be examined. The testicle may often be distinguished as an opaque mass at the back of the mass of translucent liquid. Should the light not be freely transmitted, it is probably because the fluid is rendered turbid by the admixture of blood or pus. If the fluid consists of blood, the tumor being in fact a hæmatocele, the light will be altogether obstructed.

A hydrocele can only be cured by causing the evacuation or absorption of the liquid, and the cohesion of the walls of the tunica vaginalis. Sometimes, in boys, absorption may be caused by the pressure of a suspensory bag, after the liquid has been let out; or by covering the scrotum for several weeks with lint dipped in a lotion composed of one ounce of hydrochlorate of ammonia to a pint of water, the child being kept in bed.* In adults, severer measures are usually necessary.

When the surgeon merely gives exit to the liquid contents of a hydrocele, he is said to perform the *palliative* operation. This is done with a trocar and canula. The patient stands, or sits on the edge of a chair or bed, the surgeon sitting on a chair in front of him. A vessel to receive the liquid as it flows should be placed within reach, and a little brandy and water, or other stimulus, in case the operation should cause syncope. The surgeon

grasps the tumor by its posterior part with his left hand, so as to render its walls tense in front. Now, holding the trocar and canula, duly oiled, in his right, the forefinger being applied along the instrument so as to limit the extent of its penetration, he plunges the point directly into the tumor, and as soon as the walls are fairly pierced, depresses the handle so as to avoid wounding the testis, (*Fig.* 145.) The trocar is now withdrawn, and the liquid flows out through the canula; the last

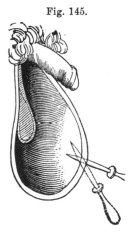

Fig. 145.

portions of it are apt to be tinged with blood, especially

---

* Forster on the Surgical Diseases of Children.

in large hydroceles, some of the small blood-vessels
rupturing as the pressure is taken off them. As soon
as the sac is emptied, the canula is in its turn withdrawn, and a little bit of adhesive plaster applied over
the wound.

When the *radical cure* of hydrocele is aimed at,
either of several plans may be chosen. That most commonly performed is merely an addition to the palliative
operation above described. The liquid being drawn off,
the canula is kept in its place until an injection is made
through it of some irritant fluid, such as wine or tincture
of iodine diluted with water. About two parts of water
to one of the alcoholic liquor will generally be about
the due proportion; the quantity must be regulated by
the size of the sac. Before proceeding to the injection,
the surgeon should ascertain that the point of the canula
has not slipped from the cavity of the tunica vaginalis
into the cellular tissue of the scrotum; since inflammation, abscess and grave constitutional disturbance would
be very apt to follow the diffusion of the irritant fluid
beneath the skin.

Some judgment must be exercised in regard to the
length of time during which the injected liquid is allowed
to remain in the cavity. Often intense pain, even inducing syncope, is caused by its entrance; and then it
should be allowed to flow out through the canula after a
few seconds. When, however, no suffering results from
its presence, it may be kept in for a much longer time.
All the injected liquid does not escape.

Should very little inflammation ensue during the
twenty-four hours succeeding the operation, the patient

should be directed to move about actively until the part becomes painful. When on the other hand the action becomes excessive, lead-water and laudanum, evaporating lotions, or cold water-dressing, may be applied to the scrotum.

Another form of the radical cure is the passage of a seton through a portion of the cavity of the sac. This plan has been preferred by some in cases of children. A few years since, it was proposed by Prof. Simpson of Edinburgh to use wire as a material for setons for this purpose; and the idea is said by some to have been found practically useful. Care should, however, be taken not to let the inflammation run too high; the seton being removed in a few days, and cooling lotions applied to the parts.

Incision of the sac, excision of a portion of its walls, keeping a tent inserted in an opening into the sac, and the application of a strong caustic, have been at different times proposed and practised in the treatment of hydrocele; but they have all fallen into disuse, the plan of injection being preferable in almost all cases, and being perfectly safe when properly carried out.

DUTIES OF ASSISTANTS IN SURGICAL OPERATIONS.

Different operators vary much in their relations to their assistants. Some surgeons prefer doing nearly everything for themselves; others confine their duties to the chief steps, leaving all the minor arrangements to their subordinates. Again, there are some operations which, for obvious reasons, necessarily involve the aid of a number of qualified persons. But in all cases, the surgeon should know exactly what reliable assistance is at hand, and should be able and willing to instruct those about him in the duties for which they will be called upon. No operator is so skilful that he may not be baffled, perhaps at a critical moment, by awkwardness or blundering on the part of a helper.

Before proceeding to an operation, the surgeon should assign to those who are to assist him the various duties they are to perform; and these duties must be strictly adhered to throughout by each one, unless in the case of some extraordinary and unforeseen emergency, demanding instant action.

Whenever anæsthetics are given, one person should have charge of their administration. He should inform himself from time to time of the state of the pulse, and should carefully watch the respiration. It is well also for him to examine occasionally the condition of the pupils.

In hospital practice, the struggling of the patient while he is passing into the state of anæsthesia is generally controlled by the hired nurses of the institution; but in private this duty has to be done by the bystanders, except in rare cases. The proper way to confine the limbs is to straighten them out; a very muscular man may require one person to each arm, and one to each leg. Pressure should be made on the knees to control the legs, and on the middle of each forearm and on the shoulder to keep down the body and the upper extremities.

Directions have been elsewhere given (see Chapter V.) for the guidance of those intrusted with the administration of the anæsthetic. I would simply repeat here, that the etherizer should stand behind the head of the patient, grasping it between his spread hands, and holding the sponge, towel, or handkerchief in place with his thumbs; the complete control of the head given by this method adds greatly to the convenience of all concerned.

Wine, brandy, spirits of ammonia, or some other stimulant, should always be within reach when any serious operation is to be performed.

Sometimes all the arrangements for an operation are intrusted to an assistant. He should see first to the preparation of a convenient operating-table. This ought to be about as long and wide as an ordinary single bedstead, and about as high as a dining-table; a firm and even mattress, laid upon it, will make it just the right height for surgical use. Most hospitals are provided with one or more such tables expressly for operating; a very good substitute may be obtained by arranging four small bedside tables close together, their long edges adjoining, and laying a mattress or a number of folded blankets upon them.

A piece of ordinary floor oil-cloth, oiled silk, or India-rubber cloth, should be so placed as to protect the mattress and bedding from being soiled by blood or other discharges. In some hospitals, sawdust is heaped on the floor to soak up the blood; but a better plan is to throw an old carpet or blanket down.

Due consideration must be given to the arrangement of the table so that the light will fall properly,* and so

---

* A skylight is best, if it can be had.

that another table with the instruments to be used may be placed just at hand either for the operator or one of his assistants.

The temperature of the room has also to be carefully regulated. No large operation can be safely performed in any place where the mercury would range below 65°; and this is especially true in cases where large joints or other cavities are opened into. In my own opinion, this is a matter which is often neglected, to the great disadvantage of patients.

All the instruments likely to be needed ought to be laid in order on a tray, and covered up until the time comes for using them. In some hospitals the room where the instruments are kept adjoins the operating theatre; an arrangement which has great advantages.

The best plan, in deciding upon the instruments to be provided, is to run over in the mind all the steps of the proposed operation, and then to think of all the emergencies likely to arise. An abundant supply of well-waxed silk ligatures, suture-needles properly threaded, adhesive or isinglass plaster cut into strips of the width likely to be called for, lint, a bottle of muriated tincture of iron or of the saturated solution of persulphate of iron, one or two tourniquets, a door key with its handle well wrapped,—all these things ought to be placed in readiness.

For amputations, it is best to provide a retractor of bandage muslin, with one or two tails; some surgeons do not commonly use this article, but it may at any time be found convenient.

Well-boiled sponges, soft but of fine texture, and of

irregular shape, about half as large as the closed fist, are invaluable in almost all surgical operations.

The part to be operated on should always be shaved, if hairy.

When a child not over ten or twelve years of age is to be operated upon, it is often more convenient to have it held in the lap of a strong assistant than lying upon a table. The child should first be wrapped in a sheet or table-cloth, confining both the upper and lower extremities; the assistant then takes it on his knee, clasping his arms around it, and controlling its lower extremities with his other leg. Another assistant may now administer the anæsthetic.

Complete insensibility having been produced, the part to be operated on may be exposed, the surgeon sitting in another chair, kneeling on the floor, or standing, as the case may be.

Certain classes of operations involve special duties for the surgeon's assistants.

In *amputations* one great object is to avoid the loss of any unnecessary blood. Hence the assistant who is intrusted with the putting on of the tourniquet should first raise the limb up, and pass his hand repeatedly along it from the distal extremity towards the trunk, with firm pressure, so as to empty it as much as possible of venous blood. The tourniquet should now be applied, so as to command the artery; this being ascertained, it should be loosened entirely until the operation is about to be begun, unless there is actual hæmorrhage to be controlled.

When the flap operation is preferred, the limb is merely steadied by an assistant while the surgeon calculates the due length of his flaps, and makes the division of the soft parts. For the circular, another assistant is generally called upon to draw the skin of the limb upwards as strongly as possible, while the surgeon makes his incision through it. Afterwards, the soft tissues, in either operation, need to be held out of the way while the bone is sawed through. Some surgeons prefer to use a retractor, three-tailed if there are two bones, and two-tailed where there is only one.

In the case of the removal of fingers and toes, an assistant should be charged with holding the other fingers or toes out of the way.

As soon as the bone is sawn through, the wound is sponged, and the operator generally brings its edges together to assure himself that he has secured a good covering for the end of the bone. Next, the wound is again allowed to gape; any arteries which are plainly seen are ligated, and then the pressure of the tourniquet is gradually relaxed so as to permit the swollen vessels to be detected by the flow of blood from them. Some surgeons pick out the vessels themselves, and have the ligatures applied by an assistant; others prefer to reverse this arrangement. Others again put the wound altogether in the charge of their assistants, only exercising a general oversight of the process of dressing.

The vessels are detected by watching for the flow of blood from them, then by a quick and firm pressure with a damp sponge leaving the surface clean, when they are instantly sought for and caught either with a tenaculum or forceps, as is elsewhere detailed. Hence the assistant who has charge of the sponges ought invariably to wring them out before handing them for use.

In some forms of shoulder and hip amputations, it is the duty of one of the assistants to catch the main artery as nearly as possible at the instant of its division, and either to compress it by squeezing the whole flap, or to prevent the flow of blood by means of the thumb applied over its open mouth, until a ligature can be cast around it.

Sometimes, where a limb has to be removed close to its junction with the trunk, there is no room for the application of a tourniquet, and an assistant has to be charged with making direct pressure upon the subclavian in the case of the upper extremity, upon the aorta, or the femoral where it crosses the os pubis, in the case of the lower. This pressure may be made either with the finger, or with the well-wrapped handle of a large door key. No one should be intrusted with such a duty who is not intelligent and careful, and strong enough to make steady pressure for a length of time. He should relieve his hand from time to time by using the other one to bear upon the artery through the fingers first applied, or by calling on a bystander to do this for him.

In *resections*, it is very commonly necessary for one or more assistants to keep the lips of the wound apart by means of metallic retractors or bent spatulas.

Another office which an assistant may have to perform is to grasp the injured or dead bone to be removed, and steady it while it is sawn or chiselled off. This has also to be done sometimes in second amputations ; if the portion of bone to be held is so short as to afford no pur-

chase for the hand, it must either be seized with a pair
of large strong forceps, (Fergusson's "lion-jawed," for
instance,) or a piece of tough stick may be thrust into
the interior of the bone so as to increase the leverage.

In *lithotomy*, as practised by most surgeons, the assistant who holds the staff has an important office. He
must strictly obey the directions of the operator, who
may desire either that the staff should be pressed upwards against the arch of the pubis, or downwards so
as to project in the perineum. To this same assistant
is generally assigned the duty of drawing up the scrotum
so as at the same time to keep it out of the way and to
render the perineum tense.

Another important matter is the securing of the patient's lower extremities. Two assistants have charge
of this, one standing on either side, facing the operator;
one knee of the patient is taken under the nearest axilla
of each assistant, who with his corresponding hand takes
a firm grasp of the foot, while his other hand is engaged
in drawing the knee outwards so as to fully expose the
perineum.

Before the introduction of anæsthetics, it was customary to fasten the patient's hands to his feet on either
side, but this precaution has now been abandoned by
many surgeons. When, however, it is for any reason
thought desirable, it may be done as follows : Take two
bandages, each 10 yards long and 2½ inches wide;
double each one on itself, and make a running noose
with the loop end. Now bring the patient's hands down
outside of his bent knees, and pass a noose over each
wrist, drawing it tight; then make him grasp his own

feet, and make with the two ends of each bandage figure-of-8 turns' around the wrist and ankle successively, until just enough is left to make a firm bow-knot or flat knot over the instep. This plan is more secure than any one with a single band can be.

Many other duties fall to the lot of assistants in surgical operations, as circumstances arise at the time. Some of these are so plain, such as holding the nates apart when piles are to be removed, that no one can miss them. Tact and experience are required, as well as a familiar acquaintance with the objects and steps of the operation to be performed, to make any one a thoroughly good assistant. Everything should give way to the accurate performance of the duty, simple and subordinate as it may be, to which each assistant has been assigned. Should anything go wrong, it is the business of the surgeon to see to it, and to direct whatever changes of plan or of detail may be indicated.

INDEX.

(287)

Norman Publishing is a division of Jeremy Norman &
Company, Inc., leading international dealers in rare books
and manuscripts in the history of medicine and science.

The following people collaborated on the production of
A Manual of Minor Surgery:

Steven Hiatt, Copy Editor
Jill Rotenberg, Project Manager
Martha Steele, Editorial Assistant
Seventeenth Street Studios, Designer

The layout was done by Donna Kelley at Zetatype Desktop
Publishers of San Francisco, using Ventura Publisher. The
type is Bodoni, a Postscript font from Adobe Systems.

Linotronic output by Pinnacle Type, San Francisco.

Printed and bound by Braun-Brumfield, Inc., Ann Arbor.

With its geometrical framework, the Norman Publishing logo
resembles the constructed letters of the Renaissance, but there
the resemblance ends. The logo incorporates the capital letter
N within an arc of the logarithmic spiral, one of the most
beautiful mathematical curves appearing in nature. It links
together the graphic arts and the sciences, reflecting the dual
commitments of Norman Publishing.

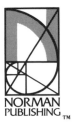

NORMAN
PUBLISHING ™